Abdeldjalil Souheil MOUMENI

Pharmaceutical compression

Abdeldjalil Souheil MOUMENI

Pharmaceutical compression

Imprint

Any brand names and product names mentioned in this book are subject to trademark, brand or patent protection and are trademarks or registered trademarks of their respective holders. The use of brand names, product names, common names, trade names, product descriptions etc. even without a particular marking in this work is in no way to be construed to mean that such names may be regarded as unrestricted in respect of trademark and brand protection legislation and could thus be used by anyone.

Cover image: www.ingimage.com

This book is a translation from the original published under ISBN 978-620-3-45209-9.

Publisher:
Sciencia Scripts
is a trademark of
Dodo Books Indian Ocean Ltd. and OmniScriptum S.R.L publishing group

120 High Road, East Finchley, London, N2 9ED, United Kingdom
Str. Armeneasca 28/1, office 1, Chisinau MD-2012, Republic of Moldova, Europe
Printed at: see last page
ISBN: 978-620-7-73756-7

Contents

In the pharmaceutical industry, compression is an operation used to shape powders into tablets. The tablet is one of the predominant galenic forms, accounting for around 80% of medicines on the world market. Its appeal lies in its ease of consumption, its variety of shapes and colours, and its ability to deliver a constant dose of active ingredient (1).

The mastery of compression technology is now well established, but as equipment has evolved over time, so has the technology itself. As a result, today's manufacturers need to understand the changes that need to be made to the process when they are about to change equipment. Given that the acquisition of new equipment, in this case tablet presses, represents a considerable investment, it is vital to get them up and running quickly and to ensure their optimum performance (2).

The aim of this book is therefore to present a summary of the research and development work carried out on the main critical compression parameters over the last few years. The aim of this work is to provide a global approach to the parameters involved in compression, in order to speed up the development of the process when a new tablet press is acquired, or when a new product is developed. This research will also serve as support for manufacturers in solving the problems currently encountered, as well as the various strategies for optimising the production of a tablet and consequently reducing its cost of production (3).

The general aspects of compression will be developed through the different mechanisms involved in this process of shaping pharmaceutical powders in order to understand the influence of the parameters.

Having established the basic principles, we will now look in detail at the different methods of compression, together with a non-exhaustive list of the main components used for compression on reciprocating and rotary machines, as well as the tooling and ancillary equipment used for this purpose.

Once these elements are in place, the third part will offer an in-depth analysis of the various parameters involved in setting up the compression process, in order to better understand their influence on the final result.

The final part will look at the problems currently encountered, such as the interaction of powders with the tooling and the various manufacturing faults, possible solutions to the problems encountered, and the impact of artificial intelligence on pharmaceutical production as a future prospect and its advantages in optimising the process in order to increase yield and productivity.

CHAPTER 1

PHARMACEUTICAL COMPRESSION: GENERAL ASPECTS

1- Introduction - Definitions

1.1- Compression

According to the European Pharmacopoeia, pharmaceutical compression is the process of compressing raw materials in powder or granule form to form pharmaceutical tablets. This operation is used in the manufacture of solid forms of medicines for easy and precise administration. Direct compression, on the other hand, refers to the process of manufacturing pharmaceutical tablets by directly compressing the powder or granules of the mixture of active ingredients and excipients, without a prior granulation step.

1.2- Tablet

According to European pharmacopeia, a tablet is defined as a solid preparation containing a setting unit of one (or more) active substance(s), obtained by agglomerating a constant volume of particles by compression or by any other suitable process such as extrusion, moulding or cryodessiccation (freeze-drying). In addition to the active substance(s), tablets generally contain one or more excipients: diluents, binders, disintegrants, flow agents, lubricants, authorised colourings, flavourings, compounds which may modify the release of the active substance in the digestive tract. When administered orally, the tablets are intended to be either swallowed, dissolved or disintegrated in water before administration. Some need to be swirled in the mouth to release the active substance. Tablets are generally in the form of a straight cylinder with flat or convex top and bottom surfaces and bevelled edges. They may bear breaker bars, an acronym or another mark.

1.2.1- Effervescent tablets

According to European Pharmacopeia, an effervescent tablet is an uncoated tablet which generally contains acidic substances associated with carbonates or bicarbonates which react rapidly in an aqueous medium to release carbon dioxide. Effervescent tablets are designed to be dissolved or dispersed in water before administration.

1.2.2- Coated tablets

According to the European Pharmacopoeia, a coated tablet is coated with one or more layers of mixtures comprising various substances such as natural or synthetic resins, gums, gelatin, insoluble inactive fillers, sugars, plasticising substances, polyols, waxes, colourings authorised by the Competent Authority, and sometimes flavourings and active substances. The substances used for coating are generally applied in the form of a solution or suspension under conditions which favour evaporation of the solvent. When the coating consists of a very thin polymer film, the tablet is referred to as a film.

1.2.3- Gastro-resistant tablets

According to European Pharmacopeia, a modified-release tablet is formulated to resist the acidic environment of the stomach and release the active substance(s) into the intestinal juice. Gastro-resistant tablets are usually prepared from granules or particles already coated with a gastro-resistant coating, or, in some cases, by enveloping the tablets in a gastro-resistant layer (enteric-coated tablets).

1.2.4- Modified-release tablets

According to European Pharmacopeia, a tablet, whether coated or not, is prepared using special excipients, special processes, or a combination of both, with the aim of modifying the rate, place or time of release of the active substance(s).

1.2.5- Soluble tablets

According to European Pharmacopeia, a soluble tablet is an uncoated or film-coated tablet intended, prior to administration, to be dissolved in water to give a solution which may be slightly opalescent.

1.2.6- Orodispersible tablets

According to European pharmacopeia, an orodispersible tablet is an uncoated tablet intended to be placed in the mouth where it disperses rapidly before being swallowed. These tablets are part of the accelerated-release drug delivery system.

1.2.7- Dispersible tablets

According to European Pharmacopeia, a dispersible tablet is an uncoated tablet or film intended, prior to administration, to be dispersed in water to give a homogeneous dispersion.

2- Operations prior to compression

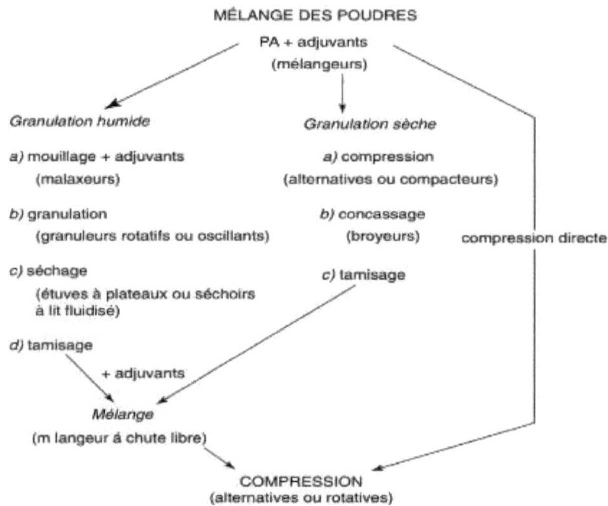

Figure 1 : The different possibilities for tablet manufacture (4)

As shown in the diagram above, except in the case of products intended for direct compression, a preliminary stage to compression is required: granulation.
The aim of granulation is to modify the texture of the mix in order to increase its density, allowing optimum flow in the matrix and minimising the presence of air between the particles. Indeed, the significant presence of air could hinder the compression process. The two most commonly used granulation methods are wet granulation and dry granulation.
Dry granulation is an operation that involves the agglomeration of powders by compressing a mixture of powders (compacting or briquetting). The resulting compressions are then crushed or ground and sieved through a sieve to obtain the desired particle size. This method is reserved for active ingredients that do not tolerate humidity or heat drying, or where the active ingredient is highly soluble in water or alcohol. This process is more complex and more expensive, particularly when the briquettes are made on alternative machines. In addition, the manufacturing process is more dusty and the wear and tear on the machines is fairly high during briquette manufacture, so the yield is better with a compactor.
Wet granulation involves the agglomeration of powders using a wetting liquid. The steps in this process are as follows (5):
•	**Mixing the raw materials:** The aim of this stage is to ensure that the active ingredient and excipients are evenly distributed.
•	**Preparation of a binder solution and transfer to the granulator.**
•	**Wetting the powders and mixing:** The aim of this stage is to create bonds between the particles, which must be strong enough to withstand the granulation process itself.
•	**Granulation:** This stage consists of mixing the powder and the liquid to obtain a granule, either by mechanical shearing or by pulverisation.
•	**Distribution of the wet granules on the tray:** This stage is specific to oven drying.
•	**Drying:** This stage reduces the humidity to an appropriate level to avoid degradation of the active ingredient and to facilitate shaping. A minimum level of humidity is required to maintain the physical properties of compressibility.
•	**Calibration: The** aim is to obtain a uniform particle size distribution by passing the granules through a calibrated grid.
•	**Addition of lubricants and disintegrants :** The purpose of lubrication is to facilitate flow and prevent sticking of the dry granules in feed hoppers and shaping machines.

- **Transfer of graded grain to a mixer.**

These stages can be carried out either in separate units, which are known as multiphase processes, or in a single unit known as an MGS (Mixer Granulator Dryer), which is known as a single-phase process (4).

For wet granulation, it's the capillary state that's of interest, as it gives the most cohesion to the mass.

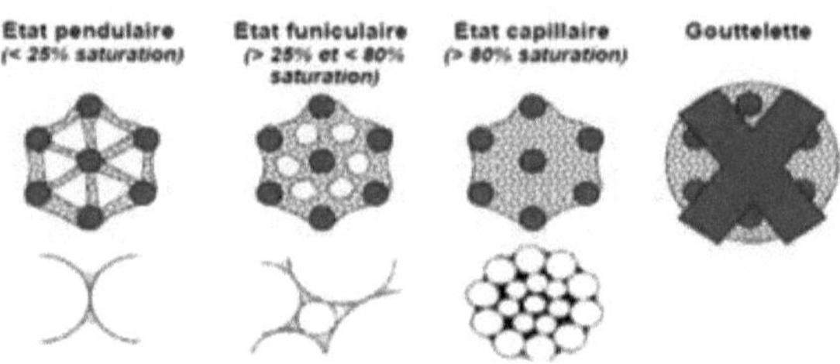

Figure 2 : Representation of the particle states during granulation Wet (6)

The advantage of good granulation is a granule with a good particle size distribution (70% granules, 30% fine particles), to ensure that the compression process runs smoothly and avoids any interaction with the equipment used for this purpose.

3- Compatibility criteria

This is the ability of a substance to give compression when pressure is applied. This ability depends on various factors which vary according to the properties of the powders used.

3.1- Compressibility

All bodies have the capacity to be compressed, i.e. to reduce their volume under the action of pressure. Compressibility represents the evolution of the behaviour of a material in response to the pressure exerted. It is an intrinsic characteristic of a body, defining its relative variation in volume as a function of the pressure applied. This value is very high for gases, low for liquids and very low for common solids (7).

3.2- Fluidity or flowability

The flowability of a powder corresponds to its ability to flow in a regular and constant manner in the form of individual particles. In industrial processes, divided solids are frequently handled, transported or stored at various stages. Thus, the flowability of powders determines the performance and smooth operation of processes, as well as influencing the quality of the final product. A powder with good flowability will flow naturally without assistance. In contrast, a cohesive powder has poor flowability, requiring the use of mechanical devices such as agitation or vibration to facilitate its movement. The dynamic behaviour of powders as they flow depends on many characteristics, which makes it difficult to express this property by a single universally applicable index. Flowability, particularly for powders composed of fine particles, is largely influenced by the intensity and nature of the interaction forces between the particles.

Moreover, flowability is not exclusively a property inherent to the powder. Depending on the speed of movement, the humidity or the surrounding temperature, a powder can behave in completely different ways (8).

There are two classic tests:

- **The funnel test:** According to pharmacopeia, 100g of powder should flow out in less than 10 seconds.

- **Suitability for settling:** The test is carried out in a settling volumenometer equipped with a 250ml capacity test tube. A 100g sample of powder is poured into the test tube, then vertical movements are applied. Several measurements are taken during this test:

- Bulk volume: Reorganisation of the powder without compacting : V_0

- Apparent volume after 10 settlements: V_{10}

- Apparent volume after 500 settlements: V_{500}

- The ability to settle is $V_{10} - V_{500}$. If the volume difference is greater than 20ml, this is a significant indication of poor flow and therefore a significant settling phase. This situation reflects the persistent presence of air between the powder particles, which in this case compromises fluidity (9).

3.3- Other properties

There are other properties that are just as important (10) :

Particle shape: This can be observed using a scanning electron microscope or an optical microscope. It influences behavioural properties such as flow, dissolution and cohesion.

Solubility: This is the volume of liquid required to dissolve a specific mass of the substance in question. Solubility increases with temperature and amorphous products are generally more soluble than crystalline products.

Moisture content: three existing types:

• **Water of constitution: This is** the water linked to the molecular formula of the substance, already present in the initial powders. It can be measured using the Karl Fischer method.

• **Water of adsorption:** This is the water present on the surface of particles under conditions of use. It can be measured by the loss on drying.

• **Free water: this is** excess water. It can be measured using an aw-meter. Water content is a parameter that influences rheological properties and density.

Hygroscopicity: This is the ability of a material to reach a state of thermodynamic and kinetic equilibrium under specific conditions of temperature and water vapour pressure. A powder is considered hygroscopic if it adsorbs a relatively large quantity of water at low relative humidity, at ambient temperatures and pressures.

Static electricity: affects physical properties and can cause :

- **The caking:** Corresponds to the creation of agglomerates and consequently disturbs the compression and flow operations.
- **Demelange:** Can cause sticking to the walls of appliances and encourage segregation.

Granulometry: This concerns the size distribution of particles. Below a critical size, particles undergo attractive and repulsive forces. They clump together on the surface that supports them when attraction is greater than repulsion. Granulometric analysis techniques include sieving, microscopy, electric field modification and light diffraction, as well as sedimentation.

Specific surface area: This is the surface area developed per gram of product. The most commonly used method is the B.E.T. method (Brunauer, Emmett and Teller), which is a mathematical model described in European pharmacopeia.

Density: This is the average mass per unit volume. European pharmacopeia distinguishes three levels:

- The true or pycnometric density corresponds to the real volume excluding interstitial voids.
- Particle density takes into account true density as well as open intra-particle porosite.
- The bulk density depends on the density of the particles and their arrangement in the powder bed.

Porosite: This is the ratio of the empty volume to the volume of the powder (11).

4- Compression stages

The basic stages of the simple compression moulding process are shown schematically in Figure 3. The process comprises four key phases:

Filling the die, compressing or loading, unloading or withdrawing the punch, then ejection

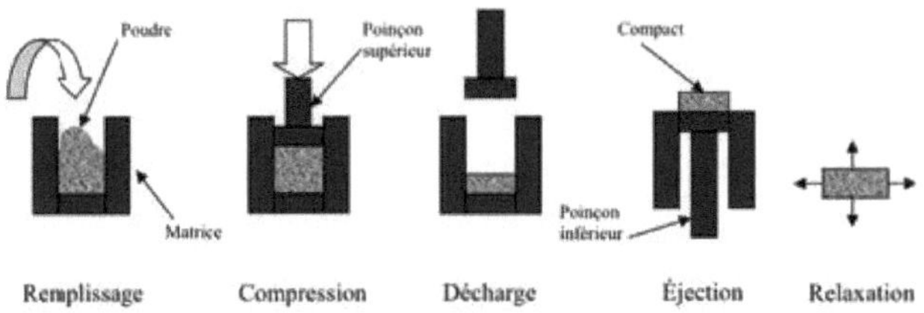

Figure 3: Presentation of the matrix compression process (12)

4.1- Filling

The die is usually filled automatically in tablet presses. The powder flows into the die and a shoe levels the powder. The flow of powder is ensured by the combined effect of gravity and the vibration generated by the shoe. Care should be taken with cohesive powders that flow poorly (in such cases, a granulation operation is often undertaken) and to ensure that when powders are mixed, there is no segregation.

4.2- Compression

The aim of this stage is to densify the powder and shape it into tablets. The top point is pressed into the matrix, and this is controlled by a set force and slice height. At the start of compression, the particles undergo rearrangement by sliding and rotation to form denser stacks (13). This flattening eliminates excess air from the powder bed and increases the number of points of contact between particles. At the end of this settling stage, the particles lose their ability to slide relative to each other, causing the powder to resist being pressed down. The particles then undergo deformation according to their mechanical behaviour. Fragile particles tend to fragment, leading to further rearrangement and greater local densification. During fragmentation, new particles are formed, starting the process all over again: rearrangement, reversible and irreversible deformation, entanglement and fragmentation to a minimum critical size (14). As for ductile particles, they tend to deform irreversibly, without fragmenting.

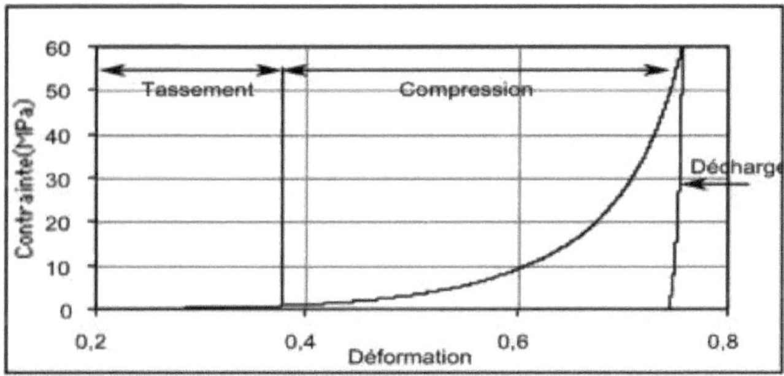

Figure 4: Typical compression curve (12)

This behaviour increases the density of the powder. During this stage, the powder gains cohesion and the pressure increases rapidly.

4.3- Discharge

During the compression stage, the powder bed accumulates energy from the various mechanisms contributing to its densification. Some of this energy is stored in elastic form, depending on both the behaviour of the powder and the parameters of the compression process, and will be released during the unloading stage (15).

This stored energy is the source of the expansion of the compact (16). During this unloading stage, it is possible for the tablet to rebound, which could cause it to delaminate (9, 12). In fact, following the withdrawal of the punch, the

The compressed powder is subjected to tensile stresses which can separate the inter-articular surfaces. As a result, depending on the properties of the powder and the compression conditions, a greater or lesser degree of relaxation of the tablet can lead to its cleavage (9,10).

4.4- Ejection

This operation is carried out either by raising the lower fist or by lowering the die. During ejection, the tablet continues to expand and is subjected to unequal shear stresses (9,10). These stresses are mainly due to friction between the tablet and the die (19). During ejection, sticking of the tablet to the walls and cleavage can occur. Figure 5 shows a typical curve representing the ejection phase. At the start of ejection, a relatively high stress is required to initiate the movement of the tablet, which then gradually decreases until ejection is complete.

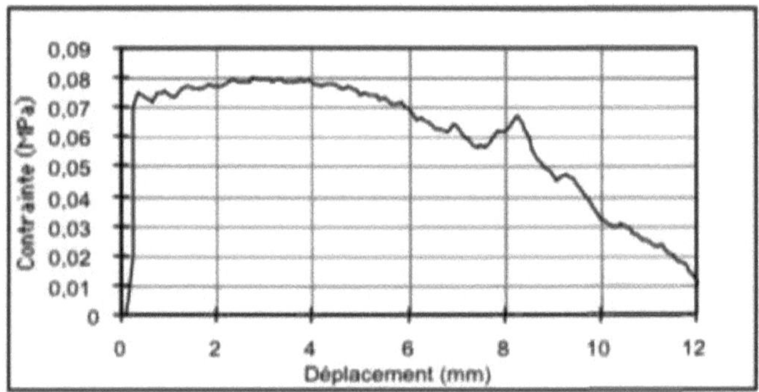

Figure 5: Ejection curve of a microcrystalline cellulose powder tablet (12)

4.5- Relaxation

After the tablet has been rejected, it continues to undergo expansion which gradually brings it to a stable state of equilibrium. However, if the powder used is sensitive to moisture or if other factors are involved, cracks may form in the tablet during this process (12).

4.6- Operation annexe : dust removal

When they leave the presses, the tablets are generally dusty. In order to remove this residual dust, several methods are commonly used, such as passing over a grid or perforated plate, or by suction (4).

Our understanding of powder compaction is still limited by the number and complexity of the stages and parameters governing the compression process. Indeed, various mechanisms such as particle rearrangement, fragmentation and reversible and irreversible deformations can occur simultaneously or successively. In addition, tablets contain not only the active ingredient, but also excipients, binders, lubricants and colourants, each of which behaves in a different way. Predicting their behaviour when mixed is proving difficult (20).

5- Mechanisms involved in compressive cohesion

Compression creates a number of contact points between particles. However, a compress will only form if bonds are established between these points. The bonding mechanisms involved in the cohesion of the compact are diverse and their importance varies according to the nature of the particles. These mechanisms have been classified according to what they induce (16,17):

5.1- Solid bridges

These bridges are built through chemical reactions, partial fusions or crystallisation.

5.2- Forces of attraction

The powder consists of an assembly of grains dispersed in a gas, generally air, where the particles remain in contact. This contact is due to gravity and interparticle attractions. These interactions are influenced by the nature of the particles and the distance separating them. In the case of a simple powder, these interactions are called cohesive forces, whereas in the case of a mixture, these forces are of an adhesive nature. Three main types of interaction can be identified:

• **Electrostatic interactions:** These correspond to the attractive forces between two charges q1, q2, at a distance of r. They act at a distance with a force F12, according to Coulomb's law (23):

F12 =

4ner

Or the universal constant $1/(\,4^{\wedge}er^2\,)$ is 9.10^9 N.m^2 /(CouZomb)^2

• **Molecular interactions:** Like Van der Waals forces, these forces act at interatomic distances of the order of 10 nm (24).

• **Capillary forces:** For moist powders containing a certain amount of water, capillary forces are most often responsible for establishing liquid bridges (22).

5.3- Encapsulation

Interparticle bonds can be formed by entanglement. The extent of these bonding mechanisms depends on the operating conditions and the properties of the powder, resulting in a kind of apparent cohesion without any physical or chemical attraction, due to the shape and roughness of the particles (10).

6- The different deformations

During a compression cycle, the particles undergo deformation and may eventually fragment as the punch sinks into the matrix. When the particles are compressed and there is no more space, they find themselves unable to move. Crushing by the pin then causes deformations, of which there are three distinct types (10):

6.1- Elastic deformation

A body is said to be elastic when it is capable of returning to its original shape. When it is compressed, it undergoes deformation, but once the force is released, it returns to its original shape, which means that the deformation is reversible. This type of deformation is not conducive to the formation of compacts (22,23).

6.2- Plastic deformation

A solid is said to be plastic when it is unable to return to its original shape. When it is compressed, it undergoes a deformation that persists even when the force ceases to be applied, which means that the deformation is irreversible. It is precisely this permanent deformation that is sought in order to obtain compressed materials, as it causes the particles to become entangled and, consequently, cohesive (22, 23, 24).

6.3- Fragmentation

Fragmentation refers to the process of the solid breaking under the application of a force. This rupture is also irreversible.

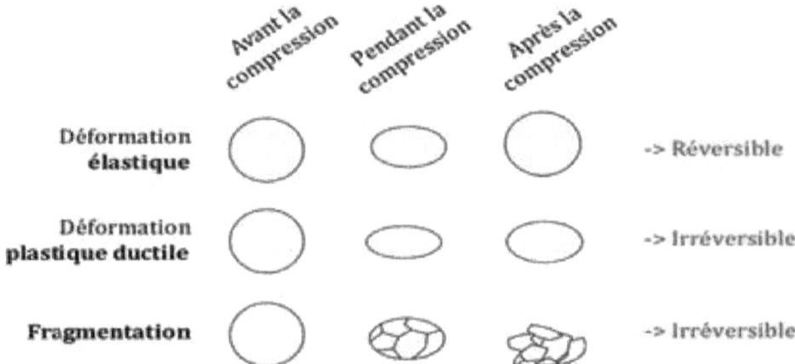

Figure 6: Diagram showing the three possible deformations after compression (28)

Figure 7 shows a stress-strain curve. The first part of the curve corresponds to Hooke's law, which gives the following linear relationship:

$$\sigma = \epsilon$$

With :

- σ : Normal stress (MPa)
- $\epsilon : \dfrac{\Delta l}{l}$ Relative deformation (%)
- E: Young's modulus (MPa) or elasticity in the case of uniaxial compression.

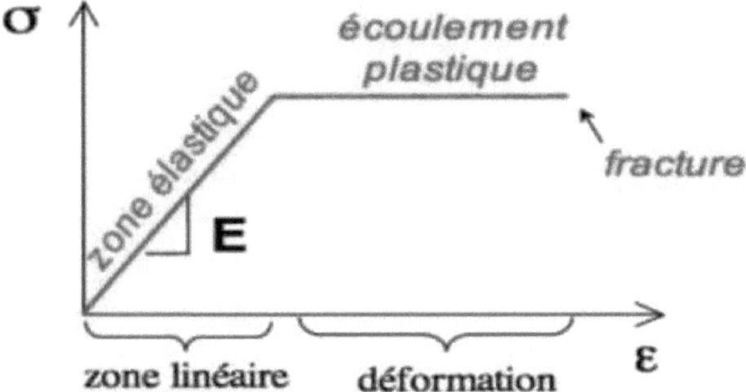

Figure 7: Behaviour cycle of a deformable solid under stress (29)

7- Special case: Direct compression

Direct compression is the most basic process used in pharmaceutical compression. It simply involves compressing a mixture of powders, including active ingredients and excipients. However, this process requires powders with specific physico-chemical characteristics. First of all, to enable the formation of a compact under the effect of pressure, the powders must be compactable, i.e. they must be capable of developing cohesion. In addition, they must be flowable. In fact, given that the process includes a quench feed system, it is necessary for the powders to be able to flow sufficiently and regularly (30).

8- Applications

At the end of the compression process, the resulting tablets come in a variety of shapes. The most common shape is round, in which case the dies are cylindrical and their diameter varies according to their unit mass. However, they can also adopt oval, square, biconvex or ovoid shapes, etc. Depending on the shape of the punches, the tablets can be flat, domed, chamfered, engraved, which allows raised inscriptions for identification, with a safety bar comprising one groove or two cross-shaped grooves, as shown in the Figure below (4).

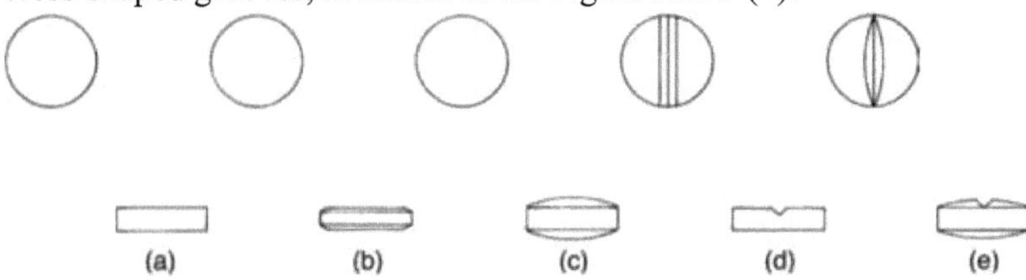

Figure 8: Different shapes of naked tablets (4)

(a) Flat tablet

(b) Press with chamfer
(c) bombe tablet
(d) and (e) : Dry tablets

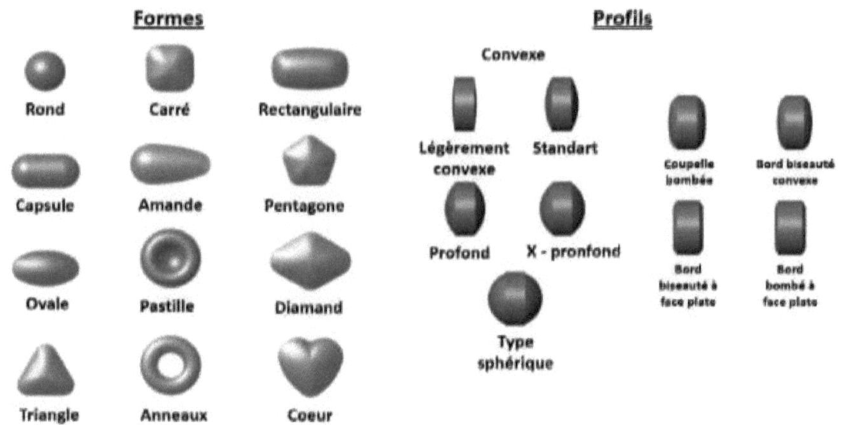

Figure 9: Different tablet shapes (31)

The tablets vary in size and mass. However, the dimensions are generally between 5 and 17 mm, and the mass between 0.1 and 1.0 g.

From a visual point of view, the main purpose of assigning colours to tablets is to make it easier to comply with treatment, particularly for elderly people who have to take a large number of medicines every day, which can lead to errors. This colour coding is also a valuable tool for the medical staff responsible for preparing and administering medicines in hospitals and pharmacies. On production sites, this differentiation helps to simplify the process of cleaning production lines, thereby reducing the risk of cross-contamination.

Since the 1970s, numerous studies have also looked at the marketing importance of tablet colours. In addition to the commercial aspect, 'psychological' effectiveness is particularly sought after, as the colours blue and green are generally the most popular.

The colours orange, red and yellow are associated with stimulating properties. For example, it is known that a sleeping pill will sell less well if it is coloured red rather than blue (31).

These tablets are then used either for pharmaceutical coating (film-coating, sugar-coating) or directly for primary packaging, where blister packs, tubes, glass, metal or plastic bottles can be used.

The advantage of good compression is that the tablets conform to the specifications required by the various inspections, but also to avoid any problems during the coating operations, such as cracks, low contrast spots, etc., and during packaging. Broken, chipped or even cracked tablets can lead to faulty packaging, resulting in an additional deblistering step or loss of product, thus affecting the final yield (32).

1.1- Tab-in-Tab tablets

Tab-in-Tab tablets represent a category of pharmaceutical tablets designed to release an active substance into the body, with a so-called lag-time following administration of the tablet, according to defined release kinetics. Belonging to the class of delayed-release pharmaceutical forms, these tablets are used in particular for the treatment of diseases with nocturnal symptoms. Their design is based on a core/shell structure, where the core contains the active substance. Tab-in-Tab tablets are produced in two different ways

compression of pharmaceutical powders. Initially, the hollow tablet is produced by conventional die compression, then a solid envelope is formed around it during coating compression, using a powder devoid of active ingredients (28).

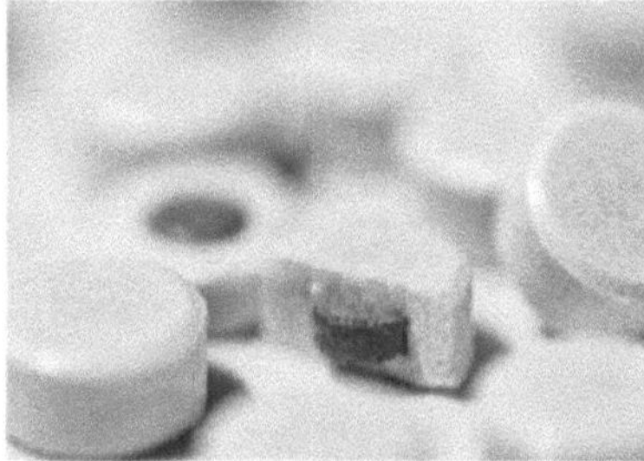

Figure 10: Tab-in-Tab tablets (28)

1.2- multilayer tablets

Some tablets come in multilayer form, usually bilayer or trilayer, which allows two or more active substances to be combined in a single dosage form. Combining several drugs in a single dose offers advantages to patients in terms of convenience, reducing the dosage load and improving compliance, as in the case of diseases requiring chronic treatment such as diabetes, hypertension, etc., but also for separating several substances.

incompatible active ingredients, or simply to control the release kinetics by ensuring a delayed effect (33).

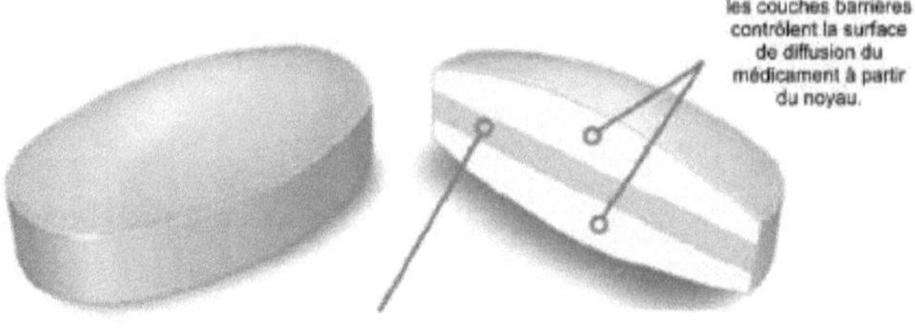

Figure 11: Triple-layer tablet (33)

The production of bilayer tablets involves sequentially compressing layers of different drug formulations on top of each other, as shown in Figure 12 . The first layer is added to the matrix and a first compression force F1 is applied. Typically, the magnitude of F1 is relatively small, as F1 is often only used as a tamping force to minimise mixing between the first and second layers and provide a uniform surface. The second layer is then added to the die, on top of the first layer, and a second compressive force F2 is applied to form the compact (34).

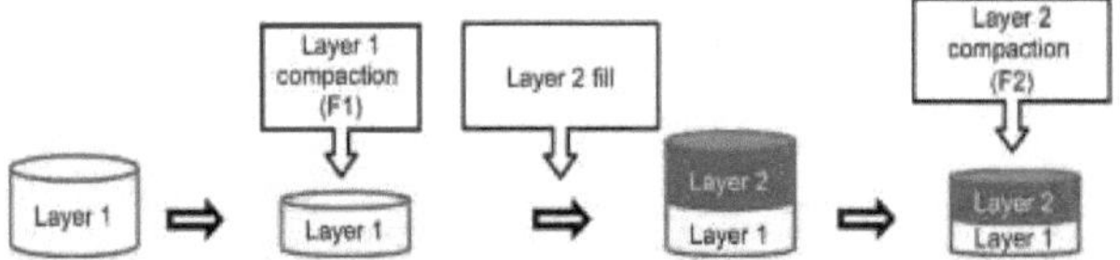

Figure 12: Illustration of the process for compressing a bilayer tablet (34)

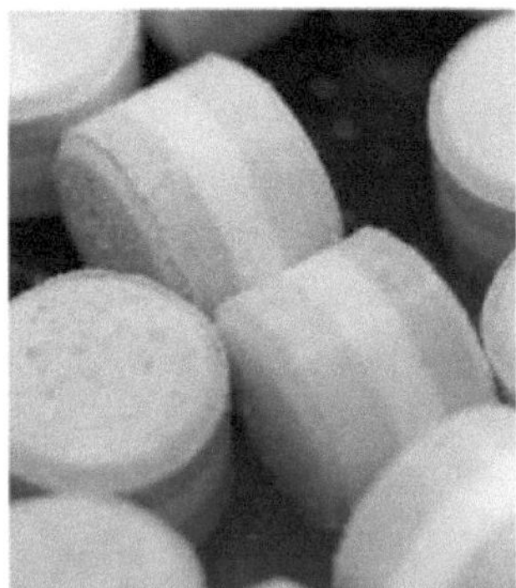

Figure 13: Illustration of multilayer tablets (35)

9- Controls on tablets

In the pharmaceutical industry, a manufactured batch cannot be released without having undergone the necessary tests to determine whether or not it conforms to the specifications. Below are the main tests carried out on a finished tablet:

9.1- Organoleptic testing

This is the first macroscopic test to be carried out visually, and enables any anomalies observed to be noted, such as :

- The homogeneity of powders
- The presence or absence of cracks
- Shine
- Rugositis
- The divide
- The colour

9.2- Pharmacotechnical controls

9.2.1- Disaggregation of tablets and capsules

This test is intended to determine the ability of tablets or capsules to disintegrate within a prescribed time, in a liquid medium and under the experimental conditions described below. A six-tank plastic apparatus immersed in a bath is used to carry out the test. Disaggregation is said to be complete as soon as all the tablet passes through the grid. Six tablets are taken from each production batch. Each tablet is placed individually in one of the tanks, and the machine is then started up, reproducing the movement of the stomach by means of horizontal and vertical movements. The desaggregation time is then measured, and must comply with the various specifications given in Table II, depending on the type of tablet (36).

Table 1: European pharmacopeia standards on tablet desaggregation tablets (36)

Tablets	Time (min)	Dispersion medium	Temperature of medium (°C)
Uncoated	15	water	36-38
Coating	60	water	36-38
Dispersible	< 3	water	15-25
Soluble	< 3	water	15-25

For effervescent tablets, the tablet is placed in a container containing 200 ml of distilled water maintained at a temperature of 15 to 25°C. Complete desaggregation of the tablet should be achieved in less than 5 minutes, resulting in the formation of multiple gas bubbles.

9.2.2- Mass uniformity of single-dose preparations

According to European pharmacopeia, 20 randomly selected units are weighed and the average mass determined. As a result, the individual mass of no more than 2 of the 20 units may deviate from the mean mass by more than the percentage shown in table 2, but the mass of no unit may deviate by more than twice this percentage (37).

Table 2: Allowable deviation for the mass uniformity of coated
or film-coated tablets
according to the European Pharmacopeia (37)

Average weight	Limit deviations as a percentage of average mass	Non-tolerated deviations
X< 80 mg	± 10%	± 20%
80 mg < X < 250 mg	± 7.5%	± 15%
X> 250 mg	± 5%	± 10%

9.2.3- Uniformity of content in single-dose preparations

The uniformity of content test for single-dose preparations is based on the determination of the individual content of active substance(s) in the units making up the sample. This test verifies that the individual active substance contents are within the established limits in relation to the mean content of the sample.

In order to carry out this test, it is necessary to assay the active substance present in each tablet. Ten units of the preparation to be tested are taken and individually dosed using an appropriate analytical method. A specific assay of the active ingredient is carried out for each unit in order to accurately determine its concentration.

The result obtained should be within approximately 15% of the average. If a value is between 15% and 25% of the average, it is necessary to carry out a new test by taking a further 20 tablets. However, none of these values should exceed 25% of the established average (38).

9.2.4- Friability of uncoated tablets

The purpose of this test is to measure the friability of uncoated compacts under defined conditions. Friability refers to the phenomenon whereby the surface of the compacts is damaged, shows signs of abrasion or breakage due to mechanical impact or attrition. The purpose of this test is to assess the resistance of the tablets during packaging, coating and transport.

In order to carry out this test, it is necessary to take a number of whole tablets as close as possible to a mass of 6.5g for tablets with a unit mass of 650mg or less. However, for tablets with a mass greater than 650mg, a sample of 10 whole tablets must be taken. Before testing, these tablets are carefully dusted.

The tablets to be tested are then placed in a rotating drum. The drum is rotated 100 times. With each rotation, the tablets roll or slide, and fall onto the wall of the drum or onto each other. In this way, they are subjected to friction and falls for a set period of time. The tablets are weighed. A loss of mass must be minimal, not exceeding 1%, otherwise it would indicate that the tablets are not in good condition.

able to withstand the handling to which they will be subjected until they are used (39).

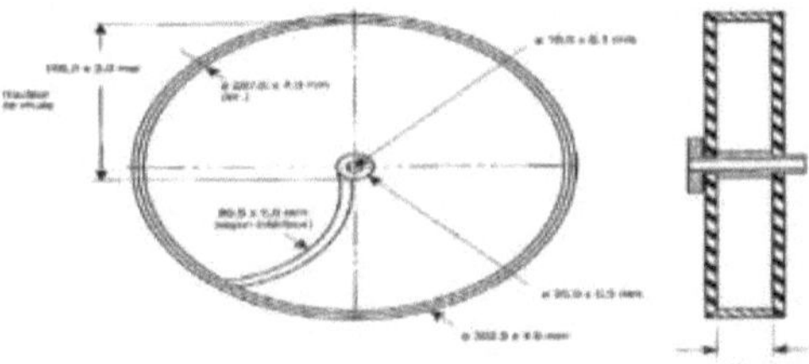

Figure 14: dimensions of the friabilimeter in accordance with pharmacopeia (39)

9.2.5- Resistance to tablet breakage

This test is designed to determine, under defined conditions, the breaking strength of tablets, measured by the force required to cause them to break by crushing.

Tablet hardness is a key parameter influencing delamination. It is therefore essential to monitor this parameter regularly during compression at regular time intervals, in order to adjust the compression force if necessary. Special devices are used to determine the minimum pressure required to break a compress. The compressed material is subjected to increasing pressure until it is crushed.

To carry out this test, the tablet must be placed between the jaws of the device, taking into account its shape, the safety bar and any engraving. For each determination, it is essential to orient the tablet in the same way in relation to the direction in which the force is applied. Measurements are taken on 10 tablets, taking care to remove any debris before each determination. The results are expressed as the mean, minimum and maximum values of the forces measured in Newtons.

The type of device used and, if applicable, the orientation of the tablets (40) should also be specified.

Note that these tests are carried out at the start of each batch, during and at the end of compression.

For in-process compression testing (IPC), each industry determines the frequency at which these tests are taken and carried out.

9.3- Microbiological quality control

During the production of a pharmaceutical preparation, whatever its formulation, it is imperative to ensure infallible microbiological quality. This means implementing appropriate measures throughout the pharmaceutical process, in strict compliance with Good Manufacturing Practice (GMP). The requirements of the European Pharmacopoeia (Ph Eur) vary according to the category of medicinal product. For tablets, which are considered to be non-sterile preparations, the Ph Eur specifies that a maximum of 103 colony-forming units (CFU) of aerobic germs and 102 CFU of moulds and yeasts per gram must be detected during microbiological testing carried out at the Quality Control Laboratory (QCL) (Ph. Eur. 2.6.12, 2.6.13, 5.1.4).

10- Conclusion

Understanding the mechanisms involved in the compression process is of paramount importance in order to be able to effectively influence the formation of compacts during powder shaping and to identify the crucial stages in this operation. In addition, a detailed presentation of the various methods of studying and controlling the compacts is of great importance, as it provides the tools needed to ensure that the process runs smoothly, both during development and during industrial production.

We will now take a closer look at the methods of compression, i.e. compression on reciprocating and rotary machines, as well as the accessory equipment and tooling for each process.

CHAPTER 2

COMPRESSION MATERIAL AND METHODS

1- Compression on a reciprocating machine

Historically, compression was initially carried out on reciprocating machines before focusing mainly on rotary machines. Although the principle is the same, it is more comfortable to describe it first with the former, which are much simpler (4).

1.1- Alternative presses

The hourly output of these machines varies from 1,500 to 6,000 tablets per hour, which limits their use to the manufacture of small batches. To develop new tablet formulas, some machines are equipped with extensometer analysis systems. These systems enable the applied forces to be measured and the displacement of the top fist to be followed throughout the various compression phases, as well as the compressibility of a powder or grain to be assessed (41).

Alternative tablet presses consist of a single station and focus on four main elements:

•   The upper and lower fistons, whose vertical movements are perfectly controlled by a system of discs and screws.

•   The die has a vertical cylindrical hole.

•   the hopper and the feeder shoe, which moves to fill, level and help eject the compact (4).

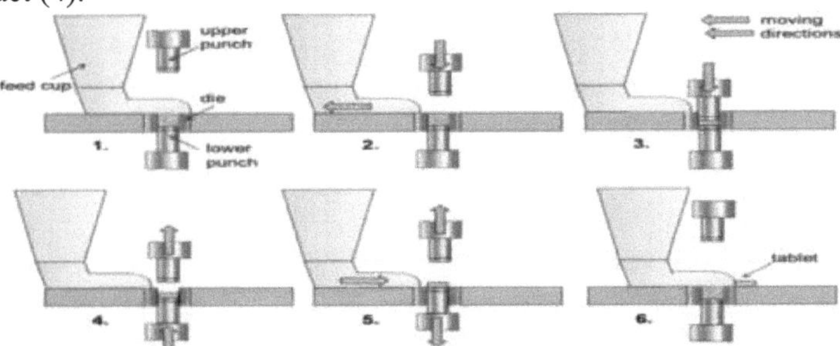

Figure 15: Operating cycle of reciprocating tablet presses showing the direction of tool movement (42)

1.2- Compression phases on a reciprocating machine

The fixed position of the lower fist determines the volume of powder to be compressed and does not change during compression. It is the upper fist that exerts the compression force and determines the breaking strength of the compact. Finally, the lower fist moves upwards and the feed shoe completes the ejection of the tablet while beginning a new filling phase. All these different phases and movements of the machine and tools are mechanically synchronised (4).

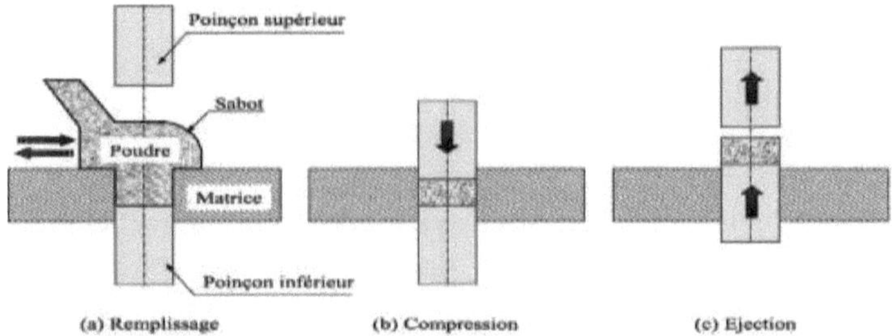

Figure 16: Different phases of compression on a reciprocating machine (43)

1.3- Advantages and disadvantages of compression on a reciprocating machine

Advantages include
- More precise tablet control.
- A wide range of tablet shapes can be produced.
- This technique is more suited to the production of small batches.
- The machines are less expensive.
- Easier adjustment and cleaning between two different productions.

The disadvantages of this method are as follows:
- Formulation constraints.
- A limited production rate and consequently low yield and profitability for the pharmaceutical industry.

It is for the reasons mentioned above (disadvantages) that the majority of manufacturers have abandoned this method of compression on a reciprocating machine, which has consequently become an outdated method (3,35).

2- Compression on rotary machines

2.1- Rotary presses

The hourly output of a modern rotary press varies between 50,000 and 10,000 tablets per hour, depending on the number of compression chambers and punches. These machines are still the only ones used to manufacture large batches (4).

Compression in rotary presses takes place between two punches, but there are significant differences when compared with alternative presses. Unlike the fixed distribution system consisting of a hopper and a shoe, it is the die and punch assemblies, arranged on a circular platen, that move horizontally. Compression takes place progressively as the two punches move towards each other. In this way, the force required to obtain the compacts is applied progressively to both sides of the powder mix, less abruptly than in the case of a reciprocating press (41).

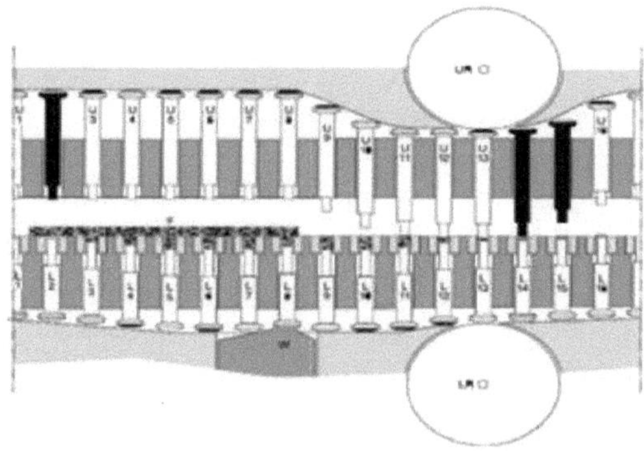

Figure 17: Operating principle of a rotary press (45)

The rotary press system is based on the use of a cam track that guides the punches throughout the process. These cams hold the upper and lower punches in position and guide them through the various stages of the compression cycle. When the press is in motion, the punches follow the path of the cam and move up and down. The volume of the compression chamber, and therefore the weight, is regulated by adjusting the position of the lower guide rail where the die-punch system passes through the filling station. Increasingly, the filling process takes place in two stages: firstly, the lower punch is lowered slightly so that the compression chamber can hold a slight overload of grain, and then in a second stage it is raised to a position corresponding exactly to the desired grain weight. The excess grain is then removed by levelling. This method ensures more even filling. Another possible improvement is to lower the lower point after trimming, so that the upper point comes into contact with the grains below the level of the matrix. This reduces powder dispersion (4).

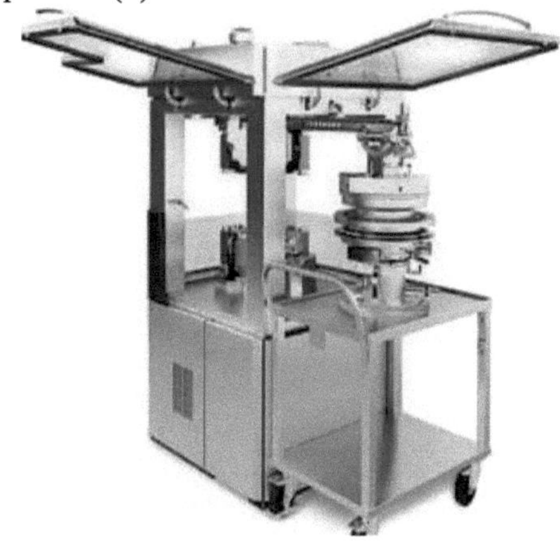

(∎

Figure 18: Example of a FETTE F20i rotary press (47)

2.2- Rotary press with interchangeable turret

With the aim of improving performance, industries are gradually adopting the various innovations proposed by manufacturers.

The aim is to reduce the time needed to change format by using interchangeable turrets. This means that cleaning can be carried out at the same time, which saves time. However, it is However, it is still necessary to clean the internal structure of the press after dismantling the turret, which somewhat limits the performance gains brought about by this innovation.

It is therefore crucial to be able to easily adjust a press to the product to be manufactured in order to optimise productivity and remain competitive on the market (48).

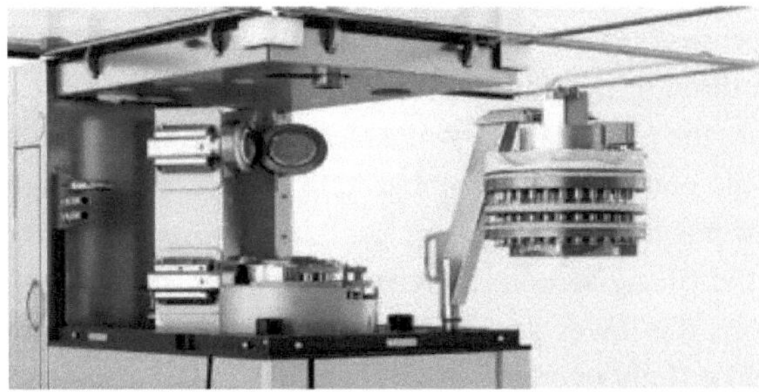

Figure 19: Rotary press with interchangeable turret (48)

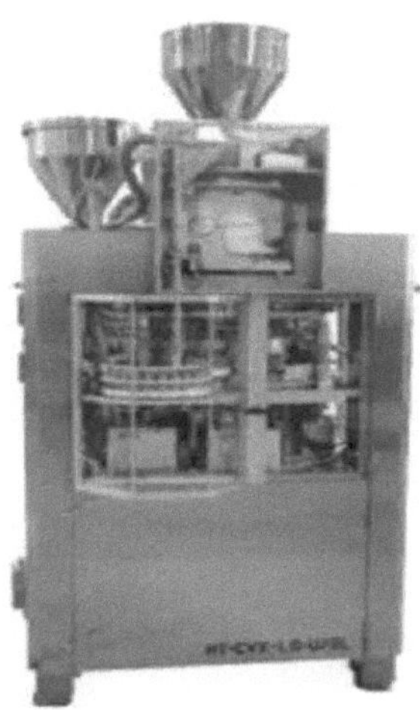

Figure 20: Example of a HATA CVX rotary press (49)

The Hata CVX tablet press, with its interchangeable turrets, expands thanks to the ability to produce tablets in two or three layers on the same machine. An exclusive sealed feed frame system, with special suction ports in front of each feed shoe, eliminates any risk of cross-contamination and ensures extremely clean delineation of tablet layers. CVX multi-layer presses can be quickly converted between single, double and triple layer configurations, without compromising either production speed or tablet quality (49).

2.3- Advantages and disadvantages of compression on rotary machines

The advantages of compression on a rotary machine are as follows:

- A very high output rate, suitable for large-scale industrial production, and consequently higher yields.
- Less sudden compression.
- Silent machines.
- Advanced automation.

The disadvantages of this machine:

- A high initial acquisition cost.
- Complex format change.
- Regular and demanding maintenance (4)

For these reasons, alternative presses are no longer appropriate for industrial-scale production. For the remainder of this chapter and literature review, we will focus on rotary presses and their various control parameters and ancillary equipment.

- **able 3** : Comparison between compression on a reciprocating machine and compression on a rotary machine

Parameters	Alternative press	Rotary press
Number of matrices	1	Up to 100
Production rate (cP/h)	From 100 to 10 000	Up to €1,000,000
Compression fist	Superior	Upper and lower
Stages of the compression cycle	Filling Shaving Compression Ejection	Filling Dosing Trimming Pre-compression Compression Ejection
Equipment	Fixed platform	Rotary turret
Benefits	Possibility of study tools for development	High production speed
	Manual filling facility	Cycle reproducibility
	Low powder consumption	-
Disadvantages	Not suitable for large batches	Useless for development because of high consumption of powders
	Unilateral compression	-

- **able 4:** Main regulation parameters for a tablet press FETTE P3030 (50)

Parameters	Description	Alert or stop criteria
Srel % main compression force	Relative standard deviation of main compression force in percent	If the actual value is higher than the set value, the green lamps flash as a warning signal, but the machine remains in operation.
Srel % main compression force	Relative standard deviation of main compression force in maximum percentage	If the Srel main compression force exceeds the Srel max parameter setpoint, the machine stops.
Individual value limit max.	Upper and lower individual value limit in maximum percentage (Main compression force in % (+ -))	If a main compression force exceeds this individual value limit, the machine stops.
Main compression force VM (KN)	The set value of the compression force required for tablet hardness in KN	-
Main compression VM max % value	Maximum average value in percent. The maximum permissible deviation from the set value of the main compression force VM is entered.	If the main compression force VM exceeds the maximum average value, the machine stops.

3- Principles of regulation

3.1- Primary regulation

The press has the ability to measure the force (or displacement) resulting from the compression of each fist. This measurement is important in the management of non-conforming tablets.

Pharmaceutical processes are not exempt from variations, and even if considerable efforts are made to control mass, it is still impossible to produce tablets of identical mass. However, in order to optimise the chances of maintaining a constant weight throughout production, tablet presses are fitted with control systems, the first of which is primary control.

This regulation takes place at the metering cam, influencing the volume contained in the compression chamber. The press measures the force generated by the compression of each individual tablet, and then calculates the average force required for compression across all the stations. Once the desired compression force value is established, the press control system treats fluctuations in force as being associated with changes in mass. The primary control loop represents the mechanism for adjusting the fill volume (and therefore the mass of the press) in response to variations in compression force, in order to re-establish the set value (51).

3.2- Secondary regulation

Depending on the variation in the mass of the presses, the secondary regulation intervenes either on the target force or on the roller spacing, depending on the technology adopted by the manufacturer. This feature is exclusive to presses fitted with in-line testers.

Automatic samples are taken, transferred to the tester by gravity or venturi, and the average weight is calculated. If this average weight deviates from the predefined mass, the press adjusts the target force or roller spacing accordingly.

For example, using "target force" technology, if the average weight measured is lower than normal, the tester prompts the press, via the PLC, to aim for a higher force. Primary regulation comes into play by adjusting the filling height, lowering the metering cam to allow the press to return to the target force. This results in an increase in the volume of pellets in the compression chamber and, consequently, an increase in the average weight.

With 'roller' technology, on the other hand, the tester, via the PLC, controls the distance between the compression rollers (a tiny variation that has very little effect on thickness but a significant effect on force). The force detected decreases, as the space between the fistons increases and the volume of powder remains unchanged. The primary control, once again, adjusts the metering cam to bring the press to the target force, resulting in an increase in the average weight (52).

4- Tools

Fistons and dies are interchangeable elements within various pieces of equipment. The interoperability of punches plays an important role in reducing costs, inventory time and variations during production expansion. Tooling can be made to measure, requiring careful model selection. The accuracy of tooling, and its wear-free condition, are of paramount importance in the manufacture of high quality tablets. The materials used, such as steel and bronze, must be strong enough to ensure long-term use. Various treatments and coatings are applied to improve their performance, particularly in terms of wear resistance, corrosion resistance and anti-adhesive properties, thus helping to prolong their service life.

A rotary machine plunger is characterised by a single mechanical part, the head of which comes into contact with the cams and the compression roller, while its active end is in contact with the mixture to be compressed. Between these two elements, the body, a cylindrical part, slides vertically in the hole in the turret, which guides it horizontally. Note: an upper fist moves with its head upwards, while a lower fist moves with its head downwards. The various components of a fiston are as follows (53):

4.1- The body

It is generally one-piece, in the form of a cylinder whose diameter matches that of the turret hole, and is perfectly centred above the corresponding die. The round knuckles are able to rotate on themselves in the turret, offering the advantage of spreading the wear of the knuckle heads in contact with the guide cams, which have a steeper slope.

However, some fistons are fitted with a guide key, either because they are not round (in which case they are called shaped fistons) and can only be centred in one position (i.e. they cannot be rotated), or because the manufacturer has deliberately chosen this type of guide, whatever the shape of the fiston.

The advantage of wedges is that the force exerted by the cam is perfectly vertical, in the same direction as the movement of the fist. With fistons of this type, the risk of seizure is reduced compared to fistons without a key, which are likely to receive an oblique thrust from their cam relative to the axis of the fiston (54).

4.2- The head

Its accentuated profile facilitates effective penetration between the cams. Usually separated from the body by a narrower section, the head is optimally housed between the cams. This feature is particularly useful for lower knuckles, which require a precise downward return, especially at the filling station. In all cases, the compression rollers exert a targeted pressure on the fist head, well in line with the axis (54).

4.3- The active part

Its diameter or shape can be precisely adjusted to that of the die. The lower knuckles have an annular undercut, which helps to release air and very fine particles during compression. The pressure of the compensator on a rotating machine is adjusted according to the diameter and shape of the active end of the fistons (54).

4.4- The permissible compression force

The resistance of the tooling to stress is linked to its specific characteristics such as the type of knuckles, format and quality. A decisive formula exists to evaluate the maximum force tolerated by the tooling, thus providing indications of the compression ranges to be avoided during production:

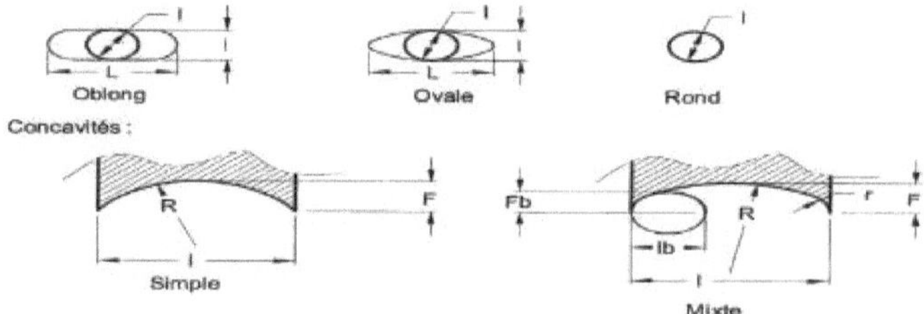

Figure 21: Maximum force tolerated as a function of the different concavities (55)

F maxi = F unit (QF) x SP

With :

- SP: Projected surface area
- F max: Maximum force
- F unit (QF): Form factor

In order to calculate the maximum force (F max) for all shapes (oblong, oval or round) and concavities (simple or mixed) of the comprimes, it is sufficient to determine the round equivalence which groups together the maximum stresses. Each contour must be simplified to a shape whose characteristics will be maximised, especially in the case of mixed concavities.

The calculation of the maximum force (F max) involves the use of several criteria, in particular the form factor (QF). This coefficient, defined as the ratio Fb / lb (or Fb = F and lb = 1 for simple concavities), is determined as a function of the actual beam and the nature of the chamfer, using the "shape coefficient" (55).

SP (projected area)

$$\frac{v <2^{L}}{1}$$

(approximate)

"SP = 0.785 xLx I   pxr

Figure 22: Illustration of the projected area SP (55)

It should be noted that the latest equipment is capable of calculating this maximum force as a function of the data entered.

1.5- Standardisation of tooling

Over time, compression tool manufacturers have responded to the strong demand for uniformity from pharmaceutical laboratories by adopting international standards. Two such standards have been developed to define standard tooling specifications, allowing interchangeability between presses and optimising the use of compression equipment (56):

- The Eurostandard, also known as the EU standard, has been adopted by member countries of the European Union (EU) as well as other countries outside the EU.
- The TSM (Tablet Specification Manual) is the standard followed by manufacturers in North America.

The demand for standardisation has increased with the proliferation of multinational pharmaceutical companies. The use of a common tooling standard for all the production sites of a laboratory has many advantages, such as the pooling of parts purchases, the ease of transferring production and the sharing of information.

By opting for a single tooling standard, pharmaceutical companies can save money by pooling their purchases of parts, thereby reducing overall costs. It also makes it easier to transfer production between different sites, as the presses and associated tooling are compatible.

With the aim of promoting the interchangeability of press punches between different presses from different manufacturers, ISO 18084:2011 was published in 2011 (57). This standard is dedicated to defining the protocols for appropriate measures aimed at guaranteeing the interchangeability of punches between different tablet presses from different manufacturers.

Despite the similar specifications of the two standards, subtle differences remain, which are of crucial importance for the correct operation of the tablet press. It is therefore essential to determine which standard is compatible with the machine for which punches are to be ordered. The major distinctions between the two standards are as follows (56):

•   In the European standard, the length of the point is 0.010 inch longer than in the TSM standard.

•   The thickness of the head is greater in the TSM tooling system than in the European Union specifications.

•   The striking heads in the TSM system have an inclined top profile (more angular), whereas in the European standard they have a domed profile.

•   The internal angle of the head for punches is 37° in the TSM system, whereas it is 30° according to European specifications.

The main difference between the UE knuckles, which have a rounded head, and the TSM angled knuckles is their impact on the passage over the rollers. This particular configuration of the UE knuckles favours a more even flow, reducing wear on both the knuckles and the machine itself. In addition, it ensures optimum contact time, favouring ideal compaction of the pellets and therefore guaranteeing the production of better quality compacts. This remarkable feature explains the adoption of the ISO standard rounded head and its use by modern machine manufacturers (56).

The figure below clearly illustrates the most striking differences between the different types of fistoon.

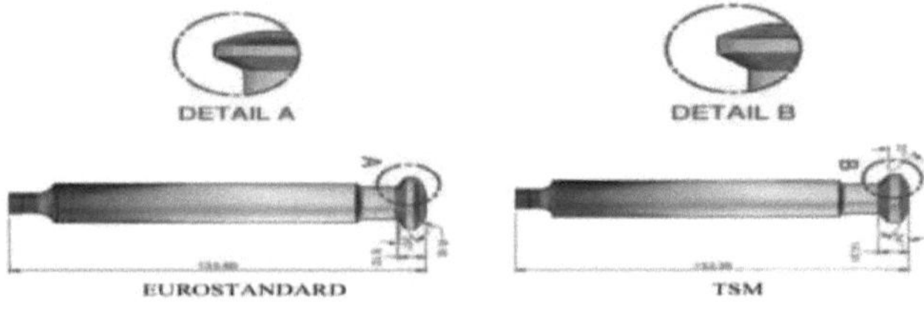

Figure 23: Differences between EU and TSM standard fistons (58)

1.6- Type B and type D fists

Two types of fist, types B and D, are widely used in the pharmaceutical industry. These dimensions were defined at the end of the 19th century by the American engineer Frank J. Stokes, who designed the first commercial tablet press. The letters B and D refer to the equipment of the time, in particular the "Stokes B1 rotary press machine" and the "Stokes D3 rotary press machine" for the manufacture of larger tablets.

During the second industrial revolution, Mr Stokes expanded his market internationally, manufacturing presses and tooling, including the "Manesty B3B" and "Manesty D3A" presses, which use similar but non-interchangeable knuckles to those made by Stokes.

In Europe, the standard adopted the dimensions of the widely-used Manesty fist, while in the United States it was the Stokes fist that was considered the standard. Despite slight differences, interchangeability between TSM and European fists is not possible, due to differences in fist head (thickness and angular shape for TSM fists, dome shape in Europe as an option for TSM fists) and fist length (European fists are 0.010 inches longer than TSM fists) (45,50).

1.7- Knuckle protection system

1.7.1- Hydraulic expansion joints

Various systems are available to compensate for compression, including the use of hydraulic compensators.

The hydraulic compensation mechanism is based on a diaphragm sphere, part of which is subjected to nitrogen pressure. This pressure, which is adjustable, has a direct influence on the force with which the roller is held. If the compression force exceeds the adjustment force of the compensator (pressure exerted by the nitrogen on the diaphragm), the compensation system acts as a damper. The roller retracts, and the compensator fist retracts (55).

1.7.2- The punch saving system

This system stops the operation of the press as soon as the upper precompression limit, which can be selected and set, is exceeded. In this way, the punch responsible for the stoppage will not reach the main compression, where the stresses would be even greater. The press then automatically moves the rollers apart to prevent the operation from being resumed, before resetting the parameters previously programmed by the production operator (60).

1.8- Tool maintenance

Tool maintenance is an important factor in ensuring the durability of punches and dies. The cleaning process is of particular significance, not only for the tooling itself, but also to avoid any risk of cross-contamination. It is essential to prevent wear and corrosion, in particular by greasing and using a preservative during storage. Lubricating the fist before use preserves and facilitates its smooth operation, optimising the interface between the tool and the press. Depending on their condition, defective knobs should be repaired, polished or replaced (61).

It should be stressed that fistons and dies are not simply inert components, but integral parts of the equipment that require regular maintenance. Their design is not only part of the development of the equipment, but also part of the process of creating new products.

5-   The rotary press simulator

Rotary press simulators, whether hydraulic or electromechanical, are distinguished by their single-station configuration. Programmable to reproduce the plunger movement profile of an industrial rotary press, these presses are very useful due to the small amount of powder required for their operation (hundreds of grams), making them particularly useful for the fundamental characterisation of materials. Because of their many advantages, these presses are frequently used in the research and development phases, as well as when scaling up production to industrial scale.

These machines are equipped with force sensors with an accuracy of 10N. Fist movements are meticulously controlled to an accuracy of less than 0.01 mm. The various sensors integrated into these machines monitor the position of the fistons and the evolution of the forces applied by the upper and lower fistons, from compression to ejection of the compressed material. An instrumented matrix can also be used to monitor the evolution of radial pressure at different stages of the process. It is also possible to adjust various kinematic parameters of the process, such as the rise time (defining the speed of movement of the punches during the compression phase), the stress holding time during compression, the descent time (defining the speed of movement of the punches during the withdrawal phase) and the relaxation time before ejection. It should be noted that several successive complete compression cycles can be applied to the same compress. In addition, these simulators allow the compression configuration itself to be modified, by performing compression with a single moving fist or, on the contrary, symmetrical compression. It is these varied settings that enable the compression simulator to reproduce the movement profile of the punches of different industrial presses (61).

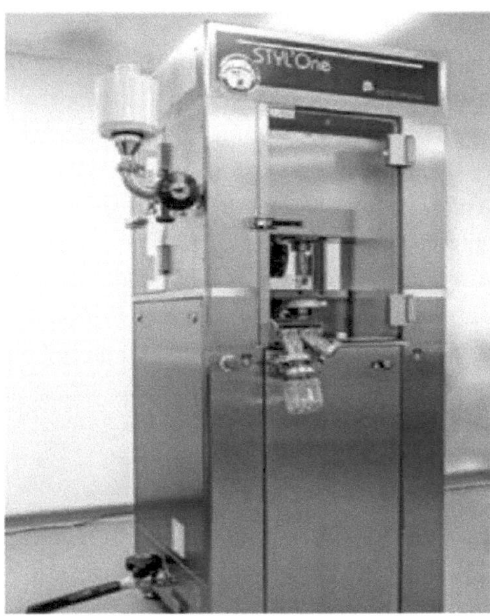
Figure 24: STYL'One compression simulator (62)

6-   Accessory equipment for tablet presses
6.1-   Metal detectors
The metal detector has a wide application in the identification and rejection of foreign body contamination. It is typically used to detect the presence of ferrous, non-ferrous and stainless steel contaminants in a variety of products such as tablets, capsules, powders, bulk products, etc., prior to their departure from manufacturing plants.

The crucial role of the metal detector comes at a precise moment when it can eliminate these types of contaminants. By automating the detection and elimination of these contaminants, it preserves the integrity of the tablets and capsules throughout the manufacturing process. Pneumatic solenoids activate the rejection mechanism, eliminating contaminants.

The importance of metal detectors in the pharmaceutical industry is undeniable. The inevitable presence of metal contaminants during pharmaceutical production cannot be completely ruled out. Metal particles, if they manage to find their way into finished products, can not only compromise later stages in the production chain, but also, more worryingly, adversely affect product quality and even lead to serious health risks for consumers. The consequences for companies include costly compensation claims and recalls, with more serious repercussions such as brand image damage and loss of consumer confidence due to impure pharmaceutical products.

The benefits of metal detectors for tablets and capsules are manifold, including the detection of ferrous, non-ferrous and stainless steel particles, the prevention of machine damage and production downtime, the assurance of product quality to the required standards, and protection against customer complaints and recalls.

The introduction of the metal detector for pharmaceutical tablets and capsules underlines its ability to detect and eliminate metal contamination, even on a small scale, in these pharmaceutical forms. It is recommended to install it after the tablet deduster in the compression line. Rejection modes are varied, allowing effective tablet rejection. Detection sensitivities are specified at Fe0.3mm and Sus0.5mm (59,60).

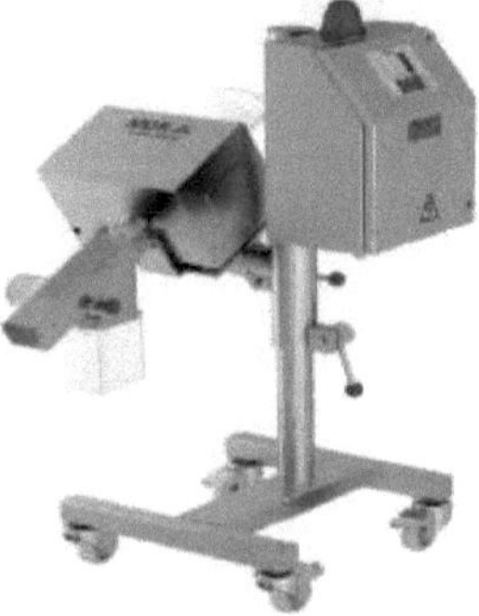

Figure 25: Gravity metal detector (65)

6.2- Dusters

It is common to see conical devices for dedusting tablets at the press exit, frequently combined with metal particle detectors. This is usually a mechanism with a spiral that guides the newly produced tablets. These compacts are raised by vibration, while a vacuum effectively removes any dust build-up affecting them (66).

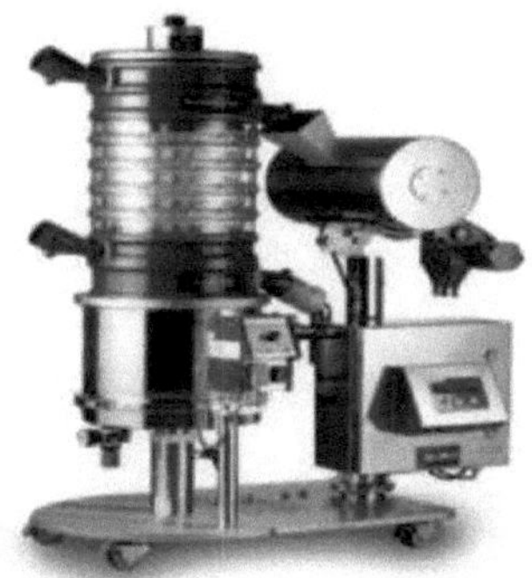

Figure 26: Tablet dust collector (67)

6.3-   PKB lubricant sprayers

PKB systems are designed exclusively for the continuous supply of dehydrating pulverulent lubricants (e.g. magnesium stearate) to a tablet press. It is an ideal system for sticky products on mould walls and punch tips while reducing the ejection force (68).

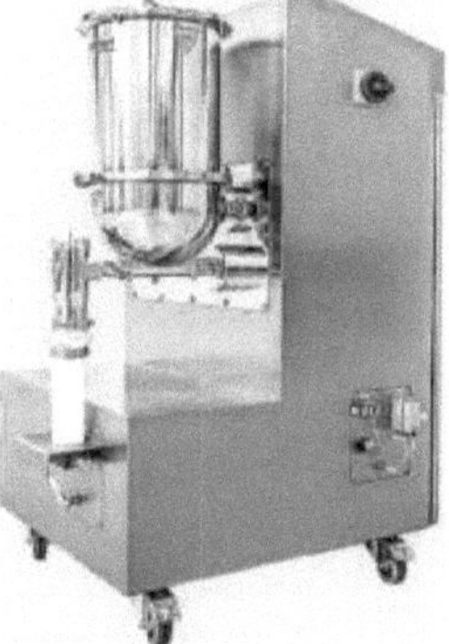

Figure 27: PKB system (68)

7-   Equipment qualification

Qualification is defined as the act of providing comprehensive documentation that the equipment or associated accessories have been correctly installed, are operating adequately and are producing the intended results. Although it is an essential element of validation, it should be noted that the qualification stages in themselves are not sufficient to validate a production process in its entirety.

The primary objective of qualification is to ensure rigorous control of equipment, thereby guaranteeing the reproducibility of processes while protecting the safety of operators and the environment. This approach encompasses all the equipment that has a direct or indirect impact on the quality of the final product. The concepts of qualification and validation are fundamental pillars in the field of quality assurance, and are imperative in regulatory terms. The qualification of equipment or the validation of processes finds its relevance in the performance of technical studies, which contribute to a better understanding of the equipment or processes by users. It also provides the assurance of control during day-to-day exploration and in the event of unexpected variations. Qualification is also illustrated by its ability to anticipate future needs in terms of the preventive maintenance of equipment, and above all to anticipate and minimise superfluous expenditure linked to possible unforeseen incidents such as breakdowns, rejections, reprocessing or repeated tests.

The investigations carried out within this framework aim to demonstrate the constant ability of the equipment to operate within the limits and tolerances previously established. This qualification process covers both the technical characteristics of the equipment and the installation and operation of all the essential components involved in the manufacture of product batches. The progression of qualification operations follows a logical and methodical sequence (69).

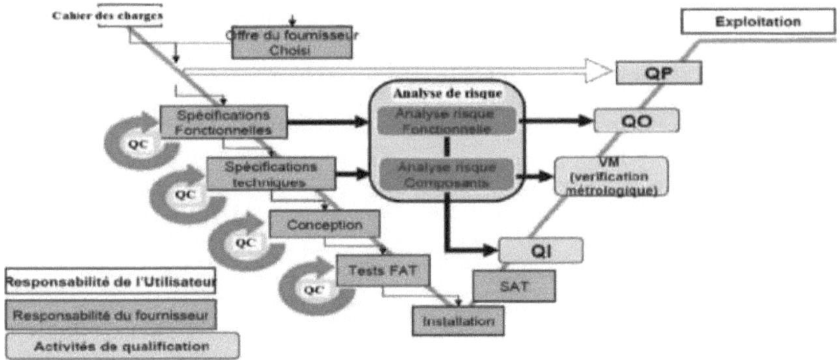

Figure 28: Schematisation of the role of qualification in an industry (70)

There are four distinct types of equipment qualification, as follows:

7.1- Design Qualification (QC)

Qualification during the design phase (QC) takes the form of a meticulous validation process, designed to provide documented proof that the design recommended for equipment, installations and systems is consistent with their intended purpose. This initial phase of qualification is an essential prerequisite. There are two types of QC:

•   Factory acceptance test (FAT): The factory acceptance test consists of a rigorous evaluation carried out at the equipment manufacturing facility. Its purpose is to ensure the conformity of the equipment before finalisation of the purchase contract or before delivery of the equipment.

• Site acceptance test (SAT): The site acceptance test is an evaluation at the equipment's actual deployment site, aimed at confirming its operation as agreed.(55,56,57)

7.2- Installation qualification (IQ)

This stage encompasses a series of checks carried out to validate the correct installation of the equipment, including the presence and correct operation of the electrical and mechanical components. This stage is carried out jointly by the engineering and production departments. It also includes metrological verification, including calibration of the equipment and re-evaluation of the compliance of the tests with the acceptance criteria (71).

When installing a tablet press, check :

• How the equipment is installed
• Checking compliance of hydraulic and lubrication circuit fill levels
• Quality assessment of assembly bridges, including joints, welds, etc.
• Validation of the conformity of the equipment's fluid connections
• Precise identification and location of parts
• Ensuring the conformity of the materials used in the construction of the equipment, paying particular attention to food safety certificates, the quality of stainless steel and surface condition reports, especially for parts of the equipment in direct contact with the product.
• Thorough inspection of safety devices, in particular emergency stop buttons and protective covers
• Validating the conformity of technical diagrams, whether electrical, hydraulic or other
• Verification of the conformity of the documentation supplied by the supplier, covering the use, cleaning and maintenance of the equipment.
• Ensuring the conformity of measurement instrument documentation and specifications

All these checks are carried out in "static" mode, i.e. without the need to run the press.

7.3- Operational qualification (OQ)

Formally documenting the ability of installations, systems and equipment to operate repeatedly and in accordance with the specifications of the product determined by the specifications, the OQ is a dynamic verification carried out outside the production phase. It follows on from installation qualification and includes carrying out dynamic no-load (or placebo) tests on each critical function, as well as calibrating the equipment (71). This stage will make it possible, for

example, to check :
- Access to functions from the press control console
- Checking the direction of rotation of the motor
- Assessment of the effectiveness of safety systems, in particular the operation of emergency stops and the interlocking of casings when the press stops
- Checking that the solenoid valves are working properly
- Calibration of measuring equipment, including strain gauges and mechanical settings
- Assessing the operation of regulatory systems

7.4- Performance Qualification (PQ)

The final stage in the qualification process, QP provides documented proof that the layout of the installations, systems and equipment allow the product to be reproduced in accordance with the pre-established specifications. Here, real production conditions are simulated using the real product rather than placebos. Each of the qualification stages (IQ, OQ, PQ) gives rise to a qualification report, listing the actions taken, the results obtained, observations on any deviations, and the necessary conclusions, with a view to making a final decision (71).

7.5- Periodic requalification (QR)

On completion of the initial qualification stages, i.e. IQ, OQ and PQ, the plant is declared "Qualified", and fit for production use. To this end, a maintenance plan specifically designed for the equipment is put in place, while a periodic monitoring programme should be drawn up and approved (71).

8- Conclusion

This presentation of the methods and main equipment used will give us a better understanding of the various parameters involved in the compression process, as well as the possible interactions with the tooling. The list of equipment is of course not exhaustive, but rather reflects the most modern and those commonly used in the pharmaceutical industry.

Following this more in-depth understanding of the different methods and equipment, we will now examine the parameters of pharmaceutical compression.

CHAPTER 3

PARAMETERS AND ADJUSTMENT FACTORS FOR THE COMPRESSION PROCESS

1- Introduction to QbD "Quality by Design

Most granules can be compressed without major problems (statistics show 70%), but the remaining 30% can pose real compression problems. Problems with tablet quality can arise for a variety of reasons. Various factors can affect tablet quality, both during the previous manufacturing processes and during the compression process itself.

The critical factors which have or could have an impact on the final quality of the tablet, together with the corresponding values generating the confidence interval, must be established and demonstrated during the validation process, and then monitored throughout the product life cycle. In order to do this, it is essential to carry out a prospective risk analysis to detect all the process factors that could critically affect the final quality of the product.

The Annex to the ICHQ8 guide describes the QbD (Quality By Design) tool. QbD provides the basis for conducting a prospective design study of a particular process and, in conjunction with the application of the ICHQ9 guide (risk analysis), proposes a procedure for establishing the optimum (reliable and consistent) design space for the manufacturing process in question.

To establish the design space, it is first necessary to define one or more critical quality attributes of the final (or intermediate) product

"CQA (74): Critical Quality Attribute. Once the quality attributes (CQA) have been defined, it is necessary to establish the factors which, during the process, have a direct impact on them, i.e. :

- Critical Material Attribute (CMA)
- Critical Process Parameters (CPP)

From this point onwards, all the tests must be carried out to establish the CMA and CPP values that confer a design space ensuring that, whenever manufacturing falls within this space, the process is reliable and robust.

1.1- The design space

Design space is an important concept in Quality by Design. According to ICH Q8 it is the representation of a "multidimensional combination and interaction of input variables (such as material attributes) and process parameters that have demonstrated relevance to quality assurance". The design space provides an in-depth understanding of the influences of the attributes (MA and PP), with particular emphasis on the critical attributes (CMA and CPP), both in terms of their mutual interactions and their impact on the Critical Quality Attributes (CQA). It is part of the knowledge space, representing the global domain under experimentation, and encompasses the control space, which corresponds to the domain in which the business process will be executed and controlled (75).

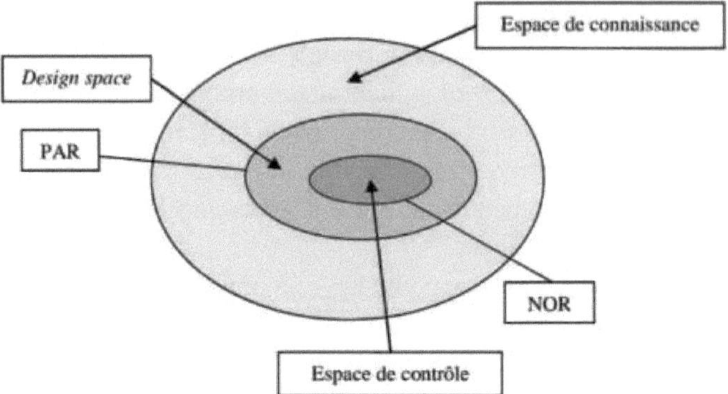

Figure 29: Interaction between the knowledge space, design space and l'espace de contrôle (76)

Design Spaces (DS) are established from the results of experiments, with their limits defined during the development project and established as the Proven Acceptable Range (PAR): a delimitation of the space within which the desired quality of the product is assured. PARs include the Normal Operating Range (NOR), representing the limits of the control space during commercial production.

1.2- Design space for a compression process

Therefore, the design space of a compression process can be summarised as follows:

Table 5: Design space for a compression process

Critical material attributes (CMA)	Critical process parameters (CPP)	Critical quality attributes (CQA)
Particle size/Granule and distribution	Type of press (model, number of stations, geometry)	Appearance of the tablet
Fine/coarse particles	Hopper design	Weight of tablet
Particle/grain shape	Feed mechanism (gravity, force feed, etc.)	Mass uniformity
Cohesive/Adhesive	Type and speed of feed frame	Hardness/ breaking strength
Electrostatic properties	Tool design (dimensions, metal quality)	Dimensions
Hardness/ Plasticity	Maximum fist load	Porosite/ Density
Actual density	Press speed	Friability

Viscoelasticite	Pre-compression force	Notable defects
Fragility	Compression force	Moisture content
Elasticity	Fist penetration depth	Desintegration
Humidity	Ejection force	Dissolution
Polymorphism	Dwell time	-

The parameters which, throughout the compression process, can affect the final quality of the compressed product can have different origins. Generally speaking, there are three main causes (75,78):

• **Formulation parameters:** These parameters are intrinsically involved in the formulation of the product, or in the selection of components (excipients and additives) and their quality.

• **Technological parameters**: These are essentially related to the equipment used. In some cases, it may be necessary to adapt to the equipment already in place, while in other situations, decisions will have to be made on the basis of specific needs, possibly opting for dedicated equipment.

• **Operating parameters:** Operating parameters are also the most difficult to set up. They include the various adjustments that need to be made to the equipment and the compression process, to guarantee optimum results.

2- formulation parameters

2.1- Characterisation of raw materials (active ingredients and excipients)

The characterisation of raw materials is an extremely important step in the pre-formulation phase of product development. Although the performance of these tests may involve additional costs in terms of time and financial resources, it is important to emphasise that the omission of these adequate tests may result in even more significant costs if the product manufactured does not meet the specifications initially defined.

The characterisation of raw materials carried out prior to preformulation is a valuable source of information which is essential in the product development process. The lack of such data would leave the formulator in a state of perplexity when it comes to solving any problems that might arise during production, during the process, or with regard to the quality of the final product. In fact, it is imperative to eliminate any potential influence of the raw materials before considering making any changes to the process variables.

In addition, these tests can also help to establish specifications for raw materials from different suppliers, enabling the most suitable product for current needs to be selected from a database. It should be noted that the vast majority of suppliers of raw materials to the pharmaceutical industry accompany their products with certificates of conformity as well as qualitative and quantitative tests attesting to the quality and purity of their products. These elements are remarkably stable from one batch to the next, and conformity tests are systematically carried out on receipt.

However, it is important to point out that information on characteristics such as the size, granulometry, shape, or specific surface area of the reviewed powder particles is often missing. However, these parameters can vary significantly from one batch to another and have a substantial influence depending on the process subsequently used (78).

2.2- Compatibility of substances

When preparing any pharmaceutical product, it is essential to ensure that the components are compatible with each other. Incompatibilities may arise, either between the active ingredient and an excipient or between two different excipients. These incompatibilities manifest themselves through various mechanisms, such as acid-base reactions or the formation of complexes, which can lead to the loss of an acid's potency, a deterioration in the product's stability, or even a reduction in its therapeutic effect. Consequently, it is vitally important to anticipate and avoid such incompatibilities by identifying possible interactions at the formulation stage (79).

The main ways of detecting interactions are essentially twofold: stability studies and chromatographic methods (78).

2.2.1- Stability studies: These are classic methods for detecting incompatibilities between components. In this approach, mixtures of active ingredients and excipients are carefully prepared and stored under demanding environmental conditions, including prolonged exposure to light, heat and humidity. It is essential that these mixtures are prepared in the correct proportions. These mixtures are then carefully investigated to detect any physical alterations. At various intervals, samples are taken to measure the concentration of the active ingredient. Signals of incompatibility manifest themselves in various forms, such as precipitation or a reduction in the concentration of the active ingredient (80).

2.2.2- Chromatographic methods: These are important tools for dissociating and characterising the different components of a mixture by generating output peaks associated with specific retention times. In practice, it is simply a matter of generating these peaks individually for each component of the mixture in question, and then checking that the same peaks are actually present in the overall mixture. When it is impossible to recover all the original peaks, and new peaks appear, this indicates possible chemical interactions that have altered the chemical structure of the products (82,83).

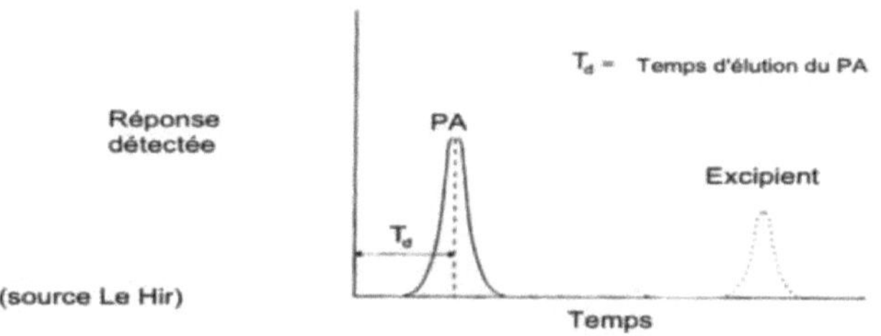

Figure 30: Chromatogram of the different peaks detected as a function of time

2.3- Excipients used in tablets and factors influencing their efficacy

2.3.1- Definition of an excipient: An excipient is a substance with no therapeutic activity, used in the composition or manufacture of a medicinal product. The functions of the excipient include improving the appearance or taste of the medicinal product, preserving its stability and facilitating its shaping and administration. It also plays a role in transporting the active substance to its site of action and in controlling its absorption by the body. Ideally, an excipient should be perfectly safe and well tolerated. However, some excipients can cause allergic reactions or individual intolerances, and are designated as excipients with a notorious effect (83).

2.3.2- Diluents: The main function of a diluent in a tablet formulation is to act as an excipient, mixing it with the active ingredient to obtain a mass suitable for producing tablets of a predetermined weight, which act as a filler.

The proportion of diluent in tablet volume is all the more significant when the active ingredients are more effective, and therefore administered in extremely low unit doses. The characteristics of the diluents are therefore of crucial importance.

It is possible to directly compress the active ingredients using a single diluent, provided that the diluent has essential secondary qualities, in particular good binding, self-lubricating and disintegrating properties.

Diluents with good compression properties fall into various categories, including lactose and its derivatives, other bones (maltose, sucrose, sorbitol, mannitol, etc.), starch and various other compounds, cellulose and dicalcium phosphate.

An effective thinner must have the following properties:

- Chemical compatibility with the active ingredient
- Ability to flow freely, encouraging regular filling of the dies in the mash tunnels
- A particle size appropriate to that of the active ingredient, guaranteeing constant dosage
- The absence of dust, simplifying handling
- A high density, contributing to better fluidity and limiting the size of the

tablet

•   Cohesion, guaranteeing the physical stability of solid forms

To choose the most appropriate diluent, compression must be studied. A simple and practical method for comparing the compressibility of excipients is to make tablets of different radial hardnesses using different compressive forces and to calculate the relationship between compressive force and tablet hardness using the least squares method. The differences in compressibility can partly be explained by differences in macroscopic structure, such as the presence of large crystals or agglomerates of small crystals bound by amorphous parts. However, for a thorough understanding of an excipient, it is necessary to move from the macroscopic to the molecular scale (73,74).

2.3.3- Binders or agglutinants : Binders play an essential role in joining particles that would not bind under pressure alone. Their presence helps to reduce the compression force required. Binders are used in two main forms: dry or, more frequently, in the form of aqueous or alcoholic solutions. In solution, binders disperse more homogeneously in the mass and are more effective.

The quantity of binder to be incorporated varies according to the specific nature of the binder and the active ingredient. Usually, the percentage of dry binder in relation to the total mass of the tablet is between 2 and 10% (84).

Commonly used binders include many hydrophilic excipients that produce viscous solutions, such as gum arabic, tragacanth, methylcellulose, carboxymethylcellulose, gelatin, starches, PEG 4000 and 6000, povidone in aqueous or alcoholic solution, as well as sucrose, glucose or sorbitol solutions.

Parameters influencing the binders :

- How the binder is incorporated : Binders can be introduced by various methods:

- Dry, followed by the addition of solvent to activate its binding power

-      In concentrated solution, with subsequent addition of the rest of the solvent, a method used to optimise the quantity of solvent in order to save drying time.

-      In solution at the required concentration, this is the most commonly used and most effective method.

The method of incorporation has a significant influence on the characteristics of the mixture intended for compression. The starch added in the external phase (dry) only has a disintegrating action, whereas in the internal phase in the form of starch, it has both binding and disintegrating properties.

In general, the use of binders in solution improves the properties of the grains more effectively than when incorporated dry or even in the presence of a solvent. Gum arabic, Avicel and carboxymethylcellulose show better wet binding properties, while PVP is not affected by the method of incorporation, and ethylcellulose shows lower wet binding activity.

- Binder concentration: Binders establish an internal matrix, thus inducing an increase in the hardness of the granules, and consequently of the compacts, in correlation with the concentration of binder present in the mix. Figure 31 graphically illustrates the crush resistance of dicalcium phosphate granules as a function of binder type and concentration. The results show a concomitant increase in crush resistance with increasing binder concentration. Notably, gelatin and starch are able to produce stiffer granules at lower concentrations, compared with gum arabic, PVP or PEG, as shown in the graph.
(85).

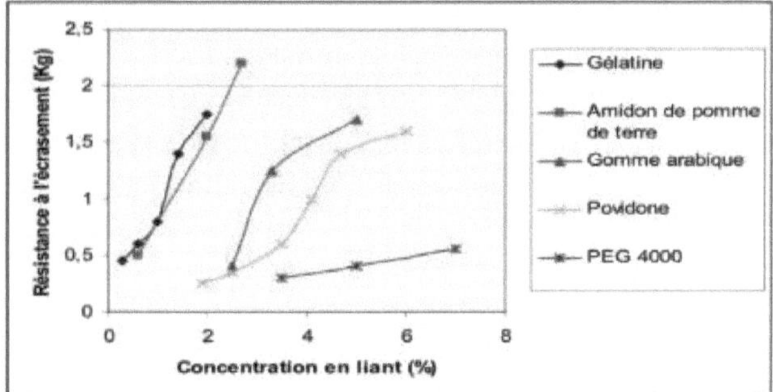

Figure 31: Variations in the crush resistance of granules as a function of the various binders present in the composition of the granule (85)

Particle size is closely related to the concentration of the binder in the mix. Figure 32 illustrates explicitly that, for all binders, increasing concentration induces an increase in the size of the lactose granules. However, a plateau is observed above a certain concentration.

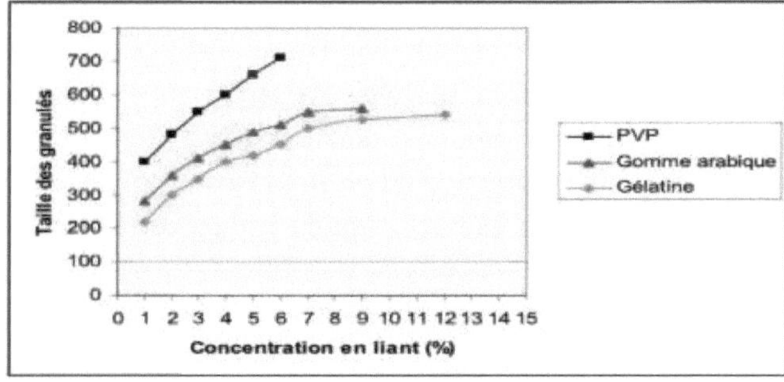

Figure 32: Influence of binder concentration and type on the size of

granules (86)
Davies and Gloor have shown that increasing binder concentration leads to a

reduction in brittleness and an increase in average grain size. However, it seems that, due to the increase in binder viscosity with increasing binder concentration, the binder distribution becomes less homogeneous, which could increase grain heterogeneity (87).

•   The mechanical properties of the binder : The mechanical and film-forming properties of the binder play a determining role in the strength and deformation capacity of the binder matrix, thus influencing the effectiveness of the binder. Healey et al (88) measured the surface tensions of gum arabic, gelatin, methylhydroxyethylcellulose, PVP and starch films prepared at different moisture contents. The surface tensions of each binder were compared as a function of moisture content. The results show that gum arabic and PVP form more brittle films, while gelatin has the highest surface tension. Excess moisture tends to reduce surface tension. PVP therefore has a high deformability due to its low surface tension, and it is this deformability that allows consolidation during compression (89).

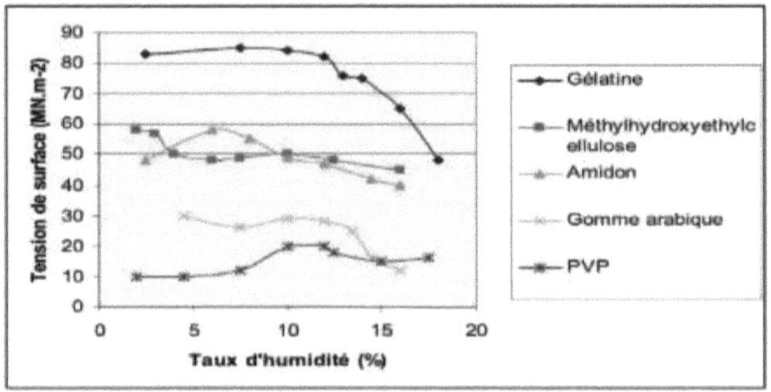

Figure 33: Influence of moisture content on the surface tension of binders (89)

In the case of cellulose derivatives, the final shape of the grains depends on the molecular weight of the chosen derivative. Herder (90) showed that low-molecular-weight derivatives produce small, compact grains, while high-molecular-weight derivatives produce large, low-density grains. It also appears that the degree of substitution exerts a similar influence to that of molecular weight.

•   Binder distribution : The distribution of the binder within the mass influences its ability to form strong, non-friable granules. Factors limiting the distribution of the granulating liquid during the wet granulation process reduce the effectiveness of the binder. For example, highly viscous binder solutions, such as starch starch, will produce more friable granules, in turn inducing the formation of friable compacts.

The process methods used to dispense the binder can also affect the effectiveness of the binder. For example, during the wetting stage, the binder is either dissolved in the solvent, and this mixture is then added to the powder mixture, or the binder is dry-mixed with the other excipients, and the solvent is then added to the mixture. In the latter case, the binder is dissolved in situ in the solvent, sometimes resulting in areas of high viscosity which can hinder the homogeneous distribution of the binder in the mass. This can lead to incomplete dissolution of the binder, which is why the addition of dry binders requires a greater quantity of the binder.

2.3.4- Lubricants : The role of lubricants in the manufacture of pharmaceutical tablets is multifaceted, although their use can sometimes have detrimental consequences on certain tablet characteristics. Lubricants are used in the manufacture of tablets for various reasons: to ensure regularity of flow, to reduce friction along the walls of the die to prevent the powder sticking to the punches, and to improve the transmission of pressure within the mass of powder (84).

Lubrication is a phenomenon that occurs when there is contact between two powders or between a grain and a powder, these elements often being fundamentally different in terms of nature, density, size, shape, structure and external surface. These components are mixed in variable proportions, according to often empirical operating conditions.

These processes aimed at improving the compression properties of the products frequently result in undesirable effects on the characteristics of the grains, more specifically the tablets. This can affect aspects such as hardness, tablet desaggregation time and the dissolution time of the active ingredient.

In fact, a study carried out by Janine Boniatti et al(91) presented different aspects of tablet adhesion to the fistons of compression machines, concentrating on glibenclamide 5mg tablets. Of the three options considered in this study, only using and refining the specifications of the magnesium stearate lubricant proved to be the most effective (increasing the hardness and drying the mix was likely to reduce productivity and lead to modifications to the already valid process). That said, the results showed that adhesion was closely linked to the characteristics of the magnesium stearate, which could be sourced from different manufacturers. The in vitro dissolution tests carried out in this study showed that changing the supplier of the magnesium stearate can influence the dissolution profile of the tablet.

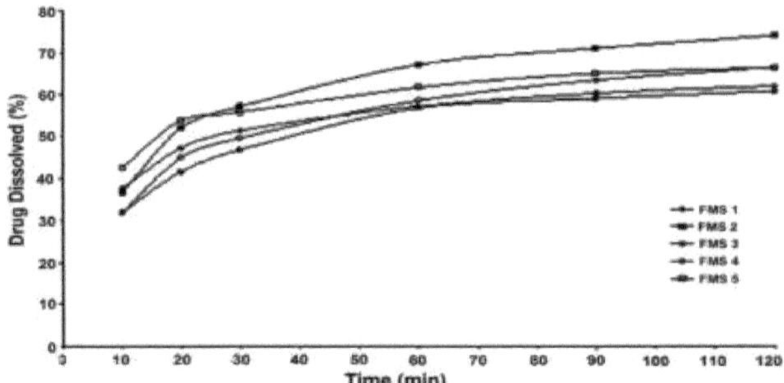

Figure 34: Dissolution profiles of glibenclamide tablets with magnesium stearate batches from different suppliers (91)

Parameters influencing lubrication (83):
• Lubricant percentage : In most cases, there is a limit value for this percentage, above which the properties of powders and tablets do not change significantly.
• Mixing time: Mixing time is a key factor. It also affects the rate at which the active ingredient dissolves when mixed with the lubricant. The mixing time has an impact on the distribution of the lubricant and leads to an increase in the lubricated surface area, governed by the equation :

$$St = Sm(1 - e^{ct})$$

• St: the separation surface at time t
• Sm: the theoretical maximum separation surface, which is a constant specific to the product to be lubricated
• C : A constant depending on the product to be lubricated
• T: mixing time.
In reality, the separation surface is a factor that affects tablet hardness, ejection, grain flow and dissolution time. Using a simple test, such as fracture toughness, it is easy to assess the impact of mixing time on tablet properties.
2.3.5- Disintegrants or desaggregants: Their role is to accelerate the disintegration of the tablet, thereby promoting dispersion of the active ingredient in water or digestive juices. These disintegrants fall into several categories:
• Those that have a different solubility to the active ingredient, for example, if they are water-soluble while the active ingredient is insoluble and vice versa.
• Those that swell in water, making it easier for the water to penetrate the compressed material and for the particles to separate. To optimise their action, they are generally incorporated dry into the mix before compression, at a proportion of 2 to 5%. Examples: carboxymethylcellulose, silica powder,

powdered starches and cellulose powder.

• Effervescent mixes, where disintegration is caused by the release of gas when the tablet comes into contact with water. This results from the incorporation of a carbonate and a solid organic acid into the mass of the tablet, generating carbon dioxide gas.

A good desintegrant must guarantee rapid release of the active substances, while maintaining satisfactory rheological properties. Super-disintegrants are new disintegrating agents that can be used at even lower concentrations than conventional starch. For this reason, any variation in their flow behaviour and compatibility must be minimised. These new molecules can be classified into three categories according to their chemical structure: modified starch (sodium starch glycolate), modified cellulose (croscarmellose) and cross-linked PVP (crospovidone) (84).

2.3.6- Various additives :

2.3.6.1- Wetting agents : In order to overcome the excessively hydrophobic properties of certain components, it is possible to incorporate surfactants as wetting agents. However, it should be noted that they can have the disadvantage of increasing the complexity of dosing the active ingredient (84).

2.3.6.2- Buffer substances: These substances are added either to protect the active ingredients from pH variations, or to protect them from hydrolysis caused by digestive juices, or to reduce their irritating action on mucous membranes. Examples: Calcium salts (carbonate, citrate, phosphate, gluconate), sodium citrate, amino acids (such as glycocol), etc. (84).

3- technological parameters

3.1- Importance of tool shape and critical control points

As previously explained, the standardisation of compression tools means that they are interchangeable between different machines on the same site.

This feature offers multiple advantages to production sites, including substantial budget savings. Indeed, as the average cost of a triplet (consisting of the upper die, the lower die and the matrix) is high, the complete renewal of a compression tool is a significant expense. Standardisation therefore makes it possible to reduce variations when changing scale. The condition of the tooling and the precision with which it is manufactured remain crucial factors in ensuring high-quality production. The process of selecting materials and coatings for the manufacture of these tools is a complex one, and must ensure that the punches are resistant to high compressive forces and abrasive or corrosive environments.

The task of selecting compression tooling is therefore of vital importance in ensuring high productivity and optimising tool life. In addition, it is essential to carry out an inspection of the various press components in order to assess the need for repairs or replacements once production has ended and the machine has been dismantled and cleaned. It is important not to wait until the next production run to detect any faults during reassembly (53).

3.1.1- Filling mode

Variations in the mass of the compacts produced, due to overfeeding or underfeeding of the product, require numerous adjustments on the part of the compaction operator. When changing materials in the tabletting machine's hopper, and depending on the flow characteristics of the powder mixtures, segregation or bridging may occur, resulting in an irregular supply of material. Consequently, it is essential to optimise the drop angles of the hoppers to ensure good flow of the mixture.

In the case of bridge formation, another approach can be used to encourage flow. If segregation is not a problem, a vibrating rod can be inserted into the mash to agitate the mixture. However, it should be noted that mounting a vibrating module directly on the mash tun can exacerbate the problem by causing product separation. Furthermore, the choice of filling shoe, also known as "**Fill-o-matic**", plays an important role in feeding the product and controlling the mass of the tablets (92).

Unlike the conventional gravity feed used in reciprocating presses, rotary presses use a force feed with different fin geometries. This alternative gives greater control over the feeding process and produces homogenous tablets of uniform mass.

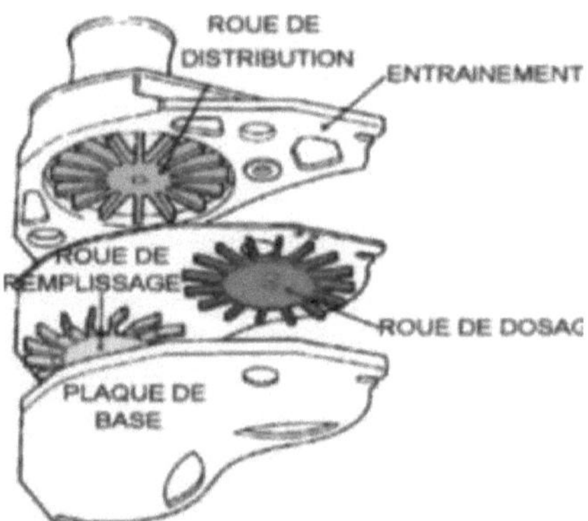

Figure 35: Diagram of a hoof shattering

power supply (93)

3.1.2- Role of the filling shoe and fins

The purpose of the rotating blades of the filling shoe is to adjust the powder flow rate according to the speed of rotation of the press, thus ensuring optimum filling of the dies and guaranteeing homogeneity in the mass of the tablets produced.

However, it is important to strike a delicate balance, as operating the filling shoe too quickly can cause disorder in the powder mix by loosening particles and compacting very wet powders, risking breakage of fragile grains.

The best approach is therefore to operate the 'Fill-o-matic' device as slowly as possible, while keeping the mass of the tablets as close as possible to the target. To study the

powder flow behaviour in the "Fill-o-matic" force-feed system of a tabletting machine, comprising three differently shaped impellers, a study has been carried out using numerical simulations (94).

In order to gain an in-depth understanding of powder flow, the authors employed a number of techniques, including the analysis of masses, particle velocities and particle segregation in the mixture. This analysis was carried out by monitoring particle colouration and calculating the time taken for particles to pass through the feed shoe.

The main results of this study can be summarised as follows (94):

•	The design of the casing geometry, in particular the arrangement of the areas containing the impellers and the different impeller profiles, has a significant influence on the particle size segregation and demixing within the feed shoe.

•	In addition to granulometric segregation, the shape of the fins plays a crucial role in the speed at which particles move, affecting the forces acting on them and shear rates.

•	A dead zone in the tremie has been identified, which could lead to compaction of the powder and cause further problems.

It has been shown that the design of the filling shoe has a significant influence on the quality of the tablets produced:

•	Firstly, the particle size segregation observed in the filling shoe is transferred to the compression matrices. This means that the larger particles, which are subject to fewer shear forces, penetrate the matrix first. The smaller particles follow, being more exposed to shear forces.

higher. Consequently, variations in the particle size distribution and properties of the particles within the matrix can lead to differences in compaction characteristics depending on their position, resulting in the risk of capping problems.

•	Secondly, segregation of the active ingredients has also been observed, which could pose problems in terms of uniformity of dosage in each tablet.

•	Finally, variation between tablets may be experienced during production due to the different distances particles travel in the filler shoe before being discharged into the compression dies. Throughout their journey through the feeder, the properties of the particles may have been altered by attrition or excessive lubrication.

3.1.3- Criteria for choosing the dosing cam

As mentioned above, the operation of rotary tablet presses is based on the principle of overfilling, where the amount of powder introduced into the die exceeds that required. As a result, the lower die is lifted to remove the excess powder. This procedure is essential to ensure a uniform tablet mass within the required specifications.

At the same time, the use of a carefully adjusted filling shoe plays a key role in obtaining tablets of uniform mass and optimum quality. The preferred approach is to operate the filling shoe and scraper blade in such a way that 80% of the powder remains in the die while 20% is pushed out. Thus, with a 10 mm filling cam, approximately 8 mm of powder will remain at the outlet (92).

If the depth of the filling cam is too shallow, this may lead to a variation in tablet mass due to inadequate overfilling of the dies. On the other hand, if the depth of the filling cam is too great, the excess material will either be ejected onto the turret plate or fed back into the feeder, depending on the type of press used. When material is ejected onto the die table, it collects around the neck of the turret and is then pushed outwards by centrifugal force, this can cause the dies to reload unintentionally after passing over the metering cam, causing a variation in the mass of the tablets. In presses where the excess mix is reintroduced into the feed shoe, it may be subjected to shear forces from the fins of the shoe, resulting in a reduction in particle size or densification which will impact on the quality of the compacts (92).

In addition, it is essential to consider the condition of the scraper blade and die cover, a critical but often overlooked aspect. These components play an important role and it is vital to monitor them. What's more, they are less expensive to replace than other parts of the press. There are different blade profiles, and it is important to note that a scraping blade with a knife edge is preferable to one with a square edge, particularly for products that tend to stick to the turret surface.

The rate at which the edge of the scraper wears is directly related to the abrasiveness of the product. It is therefore imperative to carry out regular inspections of the blade to detect any signs of significant wear. If necessary, we recommend replacing the blade (95).

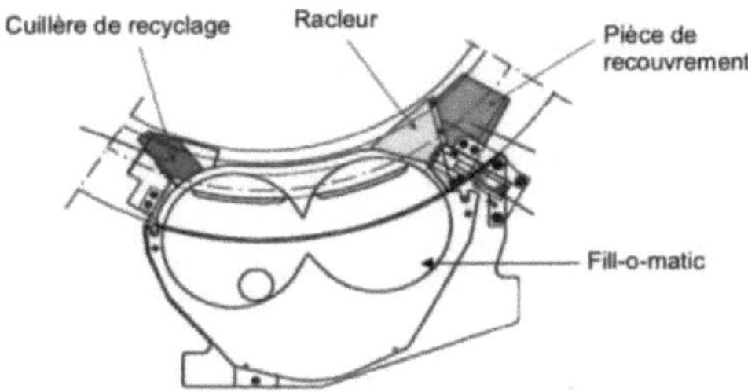

Figure 36: Illustration of the ancillary parts of the filling system (96)

The die cover plays a crucial role in preventing the product from being expelled by centrifugal force prior to pre-compression. The scraper blade is a wear-prone part, however, it is essential to note that if scraper wear occurs too quickly, this can be attributed to the condition of the turret. In fact, the surface of the turret is not always perfectly flat, and its finish can sometimes have defects. It is therefore very important to inspect these horizontal surfaces and identify the highest point. By adjusting the scraper blade according to this point, it is possible to ensure proper adjustment. In most cases, a clearance or gap of 0.05 to 0.07 mm is recommended, while the scraper springs should exert light, even pressure on the turret.

However, if the product tends to compact under the feeder, it may be necessary to raise the feeder. In this situation, it is also crucial to ensure that the dies are set at the correct depth. Dies set too high could cause rapid deterioration of the scraper blade in the first few minutes of production. On the other hand, if the dies are set too low or the wiper is adjusted too high, the powder could overcome the wiper, causing further damage to the wiper blade.

problems, such as mass variations. Careful attention to these parameters is therefore essential to guarantee an optimal production process (97).

3.1.4- Punch and die selection criteria

Punches and dies are exceptionally precise instruments, playing a vital role in the formation of comprimes.

Consequently, it is of the utmost importance to take into account the various factors likely to influence the longevity of these tools, namely :

- Corrosion caused by the action of certain products on tooling materials.
- Excessive compressive force could alter them.
- Premature cam wear.
- Damage caused by incorrect handling may result in irreparable defects.
- Internal imperfections specific to the punches, which can compromise their effectiveness.

- Overheated compression rollers or cams can damage tools.
- Inadequate lubrication of the powder mixture to be compressed, jeopardising its smooth operation.

In general, the choice of material to be compressed should determine the type of material used for punches and dies. For example, compressing abrasive materials will require special tooling, different from that used for soft, non-abrasive materials (98).

In order to make an informed choice when it comes to compression tooling, it is essential to understand the entire compression process. In most situations, dies are made from stainless steel, because of its remarkable resistance to wear. Among the most commonly used materials are the following:
- High carbon steel.
- Tungsten carbide.
- High chromium steel.

As a general rule, the ideal material should have an outstanding combination of wear resistance and compressive strength, both of which are vital for optimum performance.

3.1.5- Influence of the shape of the pins

3.1.5.1 - Conventional tablets

A study by Takashi Osamura et al (99) demonstrated that the 'Manufacturability' and 'Compactibility' of tablets on rotary machines could be reliably predicted using a formulation evaluation method that avoided tablet manufacturing failures with any shape of fist.

For all fist shapes, the properties of the presses reflected the results of pressing on a rotary machine. As shown in Figures 37 and 39, sample A, in the (III) range (poor "Manufacturability"), resulted in a manufacturing scale tablet defect (sticking). Sample D, in the (II) range (good "manufacturability"), was pressed on the rotary machine without any problems. The powders in the (II) range (poor "Compactability") were the weakest. Although samples B and C were both in the (I) range (ideal conditions), the position of sample C indicated better 'Manufacturability'. With complex fist shapes (Types 3 and 4) (Figure 38), as expected, sample C gave better "Manufacturability" and had fewer defects on the rotary machine than sample B.

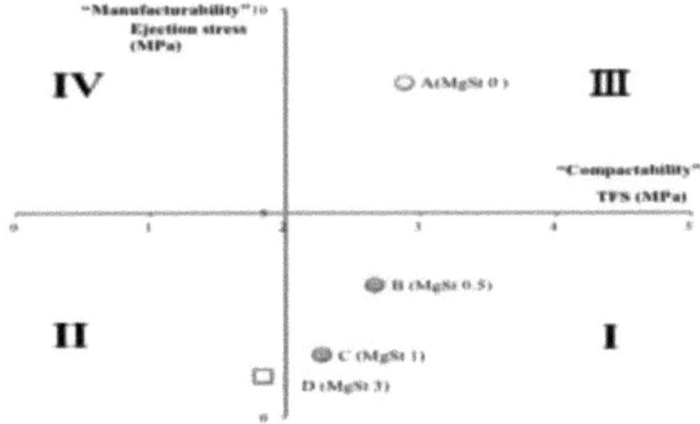

Figure 37: "Compression properties" of four formulations evaluated using the single punch tablet press (99)

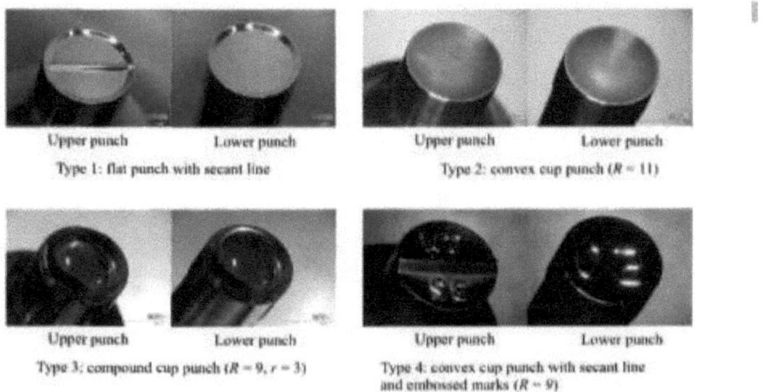

Figure 38: The four types of fistons tested (99)

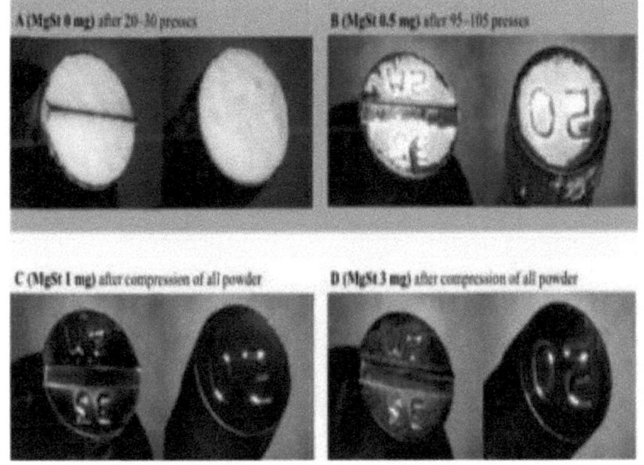

Figure 39: Adhesion of the powder to the convex surfaces of the fist (Type 4,

R=9 (99)

3.1.5.2 - Tab-in-Tab tablets

Various shapes of fist are used in the manufacture of pharmaceutical tablets. For reasons of symmetry, round punches are generally preferred when compressing Tab-in-Tab tablets.

However, it is important to note that the shape of the fist surface remains a potential variable. Specifically, the surface can be flat, flat with a chamfer, or concave, resulting in different shapes for the final tablet. Generally, the choice of fist shape is motivated by aesthetic or administration considerations, but it could also influence the compression process.

The results of this study, carried out by Leo picart et al (100), showed that the structure of the core and shell can undergo significant changes during compression. In particular, data relating to layer thickness suggest that this is linked to deformations between the layers and the shell band.

In this case, concave fistons, because of their curvature, tend to reduce the thickness of the strip more than the layer. This tendency is also observed, albeit to a lesser extent, with chamfered knuckles. Consequently, we can anticipate the effects of the shape of the knuckles on the structure and characteristics of the final compact.

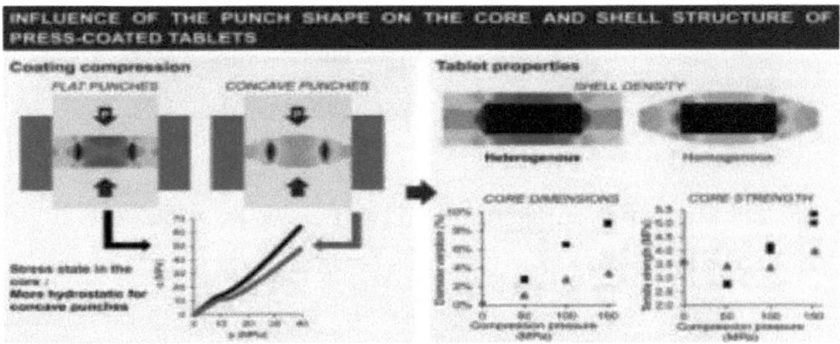

Figure 40: Influence of fist shape on Tab-in-Tab comprimes (100)

3.1.6- Fist enhancement

In order to gain a thorough understanding of compression, it is imperative to have an exhaustive knowledge of the inherent characteristics of the various materials used in the manufacture of fistons, their degree of polishing, and the many coating alternatives available. In what follows, we outline the most common deteriorations likely to occur with fistons, together with the recommended properties of steel to remedy them (53).

3.1.6.1- Premature wear of the knuckles

The essential characteristics of steel knuckles, which are essential to ensure effective resistance to abrasive wear, can be summarised as follows:

A high level of toughness.

A high volume of carbons.

Large carbide size.

Tool designers have a wide range of alloys at their disposal for making punches and dies. It is therefore essential to consult them carefully and methodically in order to determine the alloy best suited to the production required (74).

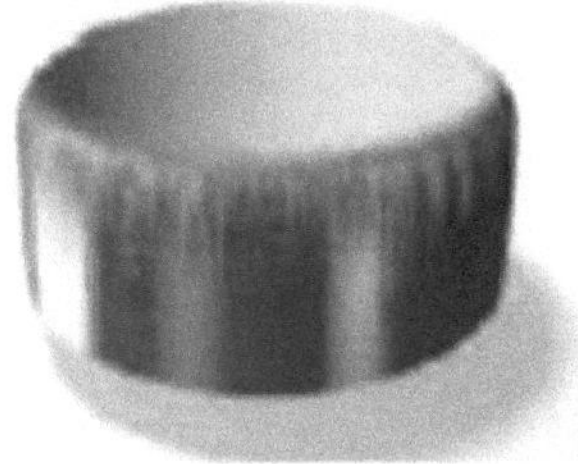

Figure 41: Use fist (74)

3.1.6.2- Active part of the ebreche fist (Chipping)

This phenomenon usually occurs when a punch has been in production for a short period of time. The failure is caused by a low fatigue cycle. Micro-cracks form on the active surface of the punch, progressively propagating until the edges of the punch break into pieces.

To improve resistance to chipping, it is necessary to work with high-ductility stainless steels (74).

Figure 42: Ebreche fingernail (74)

3.1.6.3- Plastic deformation

This phenomenon occurs when the tool has exceeded its elastic limit. The resulting plastic deformation causes alterations or damage to the tool's working surface. To increase resistance to this plastic deformation, it is essential to use steels with considerable hardness (74).

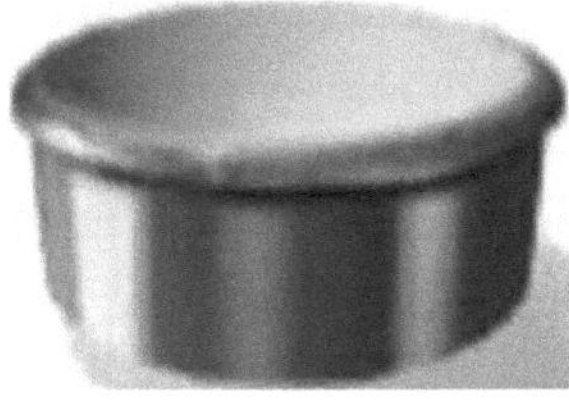

Figure 43: Deformed fist (74)

3.1.6.4- Appearance of cracks

In this context, the characteristics of the steel that guarantee effective resistance to cracking are as follows:

- Low hardness.
- High microstructural strength.

The alloy used must prevent the formation of cracks by undergoing slight plastic deformation when subjected to load (74).

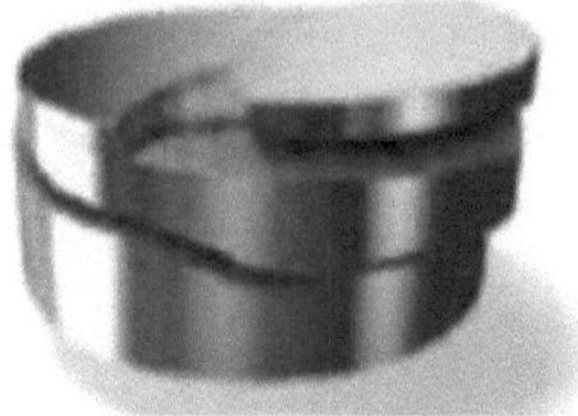

Figure 44: Cracked fist (74)

3.1.6.5- Seizure problem

The properties of steel that are of primary importance in ensuring strong seizure resistance are as follows:

- High tool hardness.
- A fairly low coefficient of friction.
- Ability to use surface treatments or coatings (74).

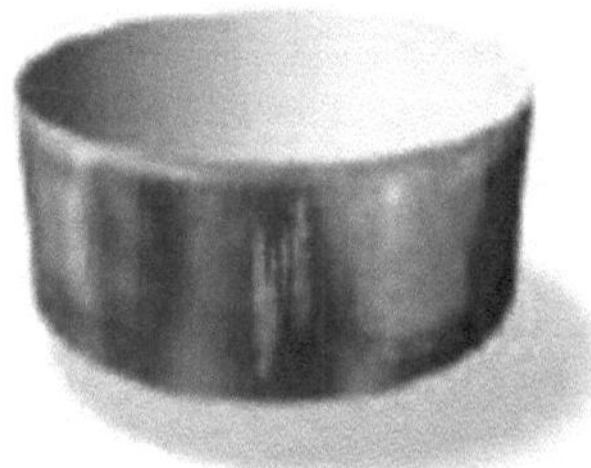

Figure 45: Influenza fist (74)

In order to prevent these various derogations, it is imperative to carry out an in-depth analysis of the constraints imposed by the product. Whether it's during the transfer of a new product or the development of another, the choice and quality6 of the materials used to manufacture the fistons will play a decisive role in 6avoiding possible future problems.

3.1.7- The different coatings on punches and dies

The main types of coating designed to improve abrasion and/or adhesion problems are as follows (74) :

3.1.7.1- Galvanised hard chrome plating

This coating is still the most commonly used to protect the surface of knuckles. It is applied by electrolysis in a sulphate bath, resulting in layers of coating around

5 microns thick. A technique almost similar to galvanising is physical vapour deposition (PVD), used for the other coatings listed below. PVD involves depositing a metal vapour on the surface of the punch. Compared with galvanising, this technique offers the following advantages:
* Improved stability of fist curves
* Preserving relief
* Optimum protection against wear and tear

As a result, it is an optimal choice for the majority of pharmaceutical tablet compression applications.

3.1.7.2- CrN (chromium nitride) coating - PVD process

The CrN coating offers a much larger surface area than that obtained by the "hard chromium plating" galvanisation process. Notable advantages include:
* Three to four times greater surface hardness
* Better performance against wear problems
* Better performance against adhesion problems
* Increased protection against wear and tear
* Value for money

3.1.7.3- TiN (titanium nitride) coating - PVD process

The TiN coating is comparable to the CrN coating in terms of performance against adhesion problems. In addition, it offers the following advantages:
* The hardness of the surface exceeds that achieved by the galvanising process by more than four times.
* Superior wear protection compared to CrN coating.
* Extremely thin layers with extremely low roughness.

3.1.7.4- DLC (Diamond Like Carbon) coating - PVD process

This type of coating takes its name from its metastable amorphous carbon nature, which exhibits intrinsic diamond properties. Applying this surface finish to fistoons generates a range of significant benefits:
* High resistance to abrasive processes.
* Long-term anti-weed properties.
* Particularly adaptable to effervescent tablets.
* A surface hardness more than six times greater than that achieved by the galvanising process.

It is also essential to note that the hardness and ductility of compression tools do not depend solely on the chemical composition of the steel, but also on its heat treatment, in this case quenching. In fact, a second quenching treatment, carefully controlled by computer and carried out at high temperatures in a vacuum environment, offers the ability to soften the material and thus prevent it from breaking.

By adopting an appropriate approach to the treatment of compression tools, it is possible to guarantee exemplary overall equipment performance. In the context of new product development or the transition between different installations, the choice of fistons requires in-depth analysis of their intrinsic characteristics (102).

3.1.8- Integrity of fistons and dies

Consideration of the condition of the fistons, and in particular their working length, is of vital importance. Variations in fist length can have a substantial impact on mass control, breaking strength and the thickness of the compacts produced. In the absence of knowledge of the specific lengths of fistons, the defects observed in the compacts could be attributed to external factors to a large extent.

It is therefore important to carry out regular maintenance and inspection operations. This is to ensure uniformity in both fist lengths and cup depths, which determine the configuration of the fist head as shown in the figure below (77,78).

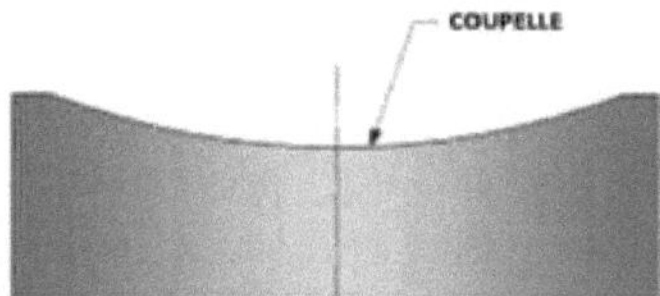

Figure 46: Influenza fist (105)

It is imperative to ensure that all fist lengths are consistent. However, the accuracy of the length of the lower fist is even more crucial than that of the upper fist. This prevalence stems from the fact that the size of the lower zone decisively determines the uniformity of the filling within the die. Thus, any alteration in this length would have repercussions on the mass and breaking strength of the compact (103).

In practice, fist length is defined as the distance between the lowest point of the active part of the fist and the flat of its head. This measurement must be within 0.02mm of the specification. Consequently, this measurement represents a critical assessment to be maintained throughout the fist's life cycle.

It is recommended that, within a set of knuckles, the difference between the effective length of the longest knuckle and that of the shortest knuckle should not exceed 0.05mm. With this in mind, it is advisable to examine the effective lengths of new knuckles added to a pre-existing assembly, in order to remain within this tolerance. If this measurement remains consistent, the new tool should perform ideally 95% of the time (103).

During the production phase, there is a direct link between punch length and compression force. In fact, the useful length of the punch can have an impact on the press force control system. As explained above, this system allows automatic adjustment of the press weight during production, without the need for operator intervention (104).

Inadequate tool tolerances will therefore affect the measured compression forces, causing the control system to respond to a variation in tool length rather than an actual variation in the mass of the compression (104).

Careful accuracy of fist length is therefore of paramount importance in ensuring consistent production in terms of tablet volume at each station, and thus effective control of process forces. However, it should be noted that, in most cases, damaged equipment results from inadequate compression of the powders. Typically, these errors are the result of mixtures requiring excessive compression forces, ejection forces that are too pronounced, insufficient lubrication or poor dust removal.

The compression press can be likened to a report card, revealing the errors of the previous stages (106).

Finally, effective lubrication of the punches will maximise their life and minimise the problems that can arise during compression. Operators should therefore pay particular attention to stopping the press when fine particles accumulate and fist lubrication decreases. Once fist lubrication is under control, there is another area that should be closely monitored: the integrity of the seals around the fists at the fist guides (the part of the turret into which the fists are inserted). Damaged seals could lead to excessive oil leakage, combined with powder contamination, which could contaminate the pellets. The collection cups at the ends of the fistons are the final barrier against this problem. When assembling and dismantling the device, their integrity should be checked (77,78).

3.1.9- Geometry of the active head of the pointer

The design of the compression tool can affect the compression process. The active parts of the fistons, which are located at the base of the fistons and come into direct contact with the powder, are of paramount importance in the compacting device. There is no doubt that these areas undergo considerable adaptation within the compression equipment. Indeed, the study of the geometry of the active heads of the punches is a particularly demanding area of investigation in the context of the advances made in the design of compression presses.

In this development, the objective is invariably to improve the efficiency of the compression process, while addressing the specific problems faced by production facilities.

As evidence of this, research carried out in 2017 looked at the effects of modifying the contour of the fist surface and the characteristics of the pellets. To achieve this, a comparison was made between the production of comprimes using two fistoon varieties, differing in the configuration of their active part. The first was characterised by an angled surface (A), while the second had a radial face (B).

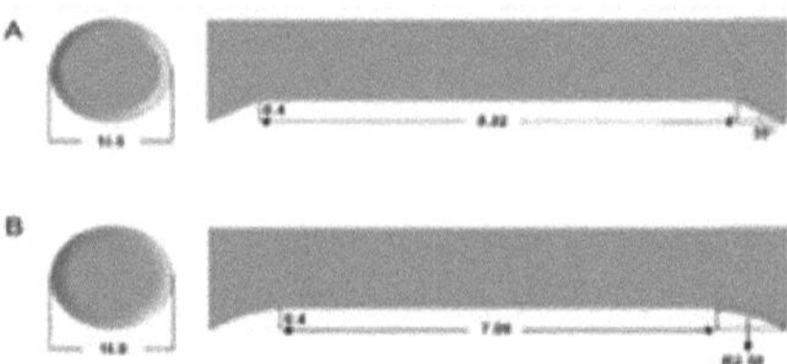

Figure 47: Schematic representation of the active heads of fistons (107)

The conclusions of this study highlighted that the adoption of fistons with a face configuration featuring a radial edge (B) presented a considerable advantage for tablet production. This approach favoured better densification of the powder, leading to an improvement in the mechanical strength of the compacts produced, while reducing the tendency to cleavage (107).

Modifying the angular edge of the bevelled surface into a curved contour specific to the radial face would allow deeper penetration of the fist into the matrix cavity during the compression cycle. As a result, greater densification of the compact would be achieved.

In addition, this curvature would favour a more homogeneous distribution of the compressive force throughout the compacted structure, which would reduce the formation of zones subject to localised stresses and consequently reduce the elastic expansion of the compact during the decompression phase (107).

3.1.10- Geometry of the fist's passive head

Over the years, the design characteristics of fistons intended for compression have been the subject of numerous adjustments aimed at perfecting the compression process, improving the quality of the finished product and increasing the durability of the instruments. In addition to the improvements made to the active heads of the fistons, the upper part of the fistons, in contact with the compression rollers, has also been the focus of numerous studies. This component of the fist is often referred to as the passive head. Head Flat (HF) and Head Radius (HR), as shown in Figure 49, can be subject to modification by tool manufacturers in order to extend tool life, improve compression efficiency and, more specifically, enhance the physical properties of the resulting compacts.

The concept of the (flat of the head) or HF of the fist refers to the flat surface of the head that will come into contact with the compression roller, and therefore govern the period of contact known as the (compression time) or (dwell time).

This period corresponds to the time during which the minimum distance between the fists is maintained (108).

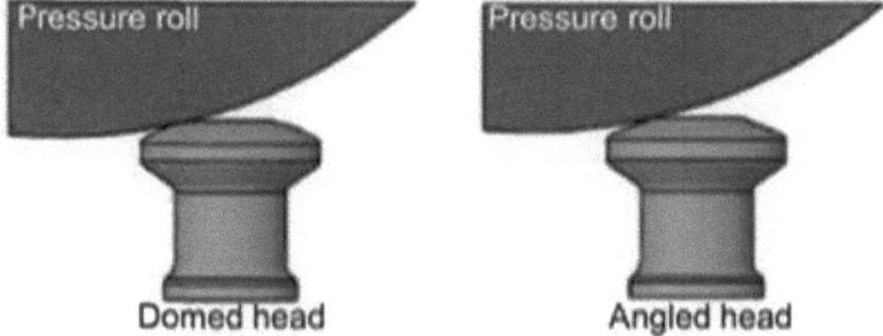

Figure 48: Schematic representation of the passive heads of fistons (104)

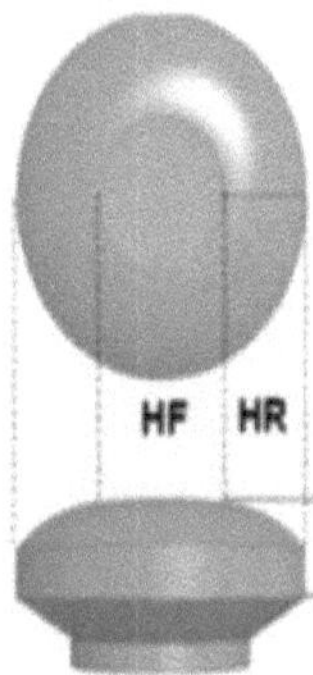

Figure 49: Diagram of a fist head (108)

The value of the dwell time has a significant influence on the behavioural properties of the powders subjected to it. A short dwell time, such as when increasing press speed, may appear to favour phenomena such as cleavage, since the dwell time is insufficient to allow complete absorption of the energy by the compact before decompression (109).

In the majority of circumstances, it is generally preferable to opt for a domed head rather than a bevelled head, as the former can help prevent cleavage. In fact, the compression roller comes into contact with the domed part earlier, which places it at a greater distance from the surface.

away from the flat surface. This prerequisite allows the air to be evacuated more efficiently before starting the full compression. The domed head configuration thus reduces the impact of the shock and limits the amount of energy to be evacuated during ejection (103).

3.1.11-Customised tooling

Tooling customisation depends on the type of tabletting machine and the desired end product, with several customisation points to consider (52). The punches and die play a decisive role in defining the shape, dimensions, marking and security of the tablet. It is essential to design the engraving font in such a way as to eliminate sharp edges, as illustrated in the figures below.

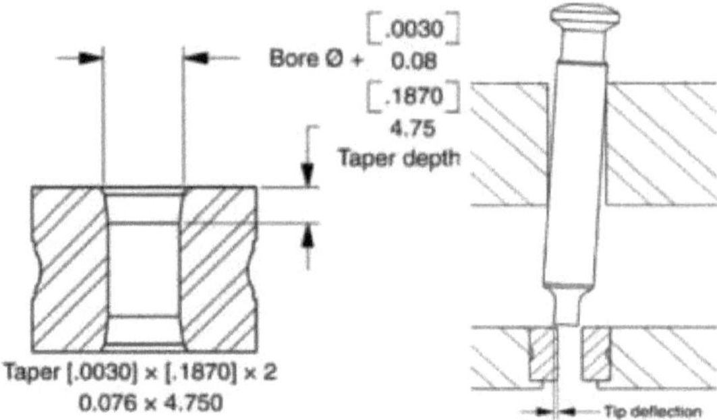

Figure 50: Example of a tapered die and a desaxial fist (110)

The engraving configuration must take into account the amount of engraving in relation to the size and shape of the tablet, as well as the characteristics of the final product. Conical dies offer advantages such as the expulsion of air at the start of compression and the possibility of turning the die upside down in the event of a defect on the upper face.

The fist key is essential for aligning the upper fist, particularly with recent, very fast-rotating rotary presses, to avoid the risk of the fist becoming misaligned.

In the context of high-speed rotary machines, the use of dome-shaped fist heads reduces the impact between the compression roller and the head of the fist, ensuring smoother transmission of force to the compression cycle. This reduces stress and the risk of premature wear on the compression rollers. The width of the fist head influences the compression time, with a wider fist head resulting in greater efficiency and reduced compression forces. However, the difference between the head and body diameters increases the risk of tool fracture (110).

In the case of the manufacture of small tablets, the use of multipoint punches makes it possible to increase production capacity at lower cost, as does the use of various systems for securing the points (111).

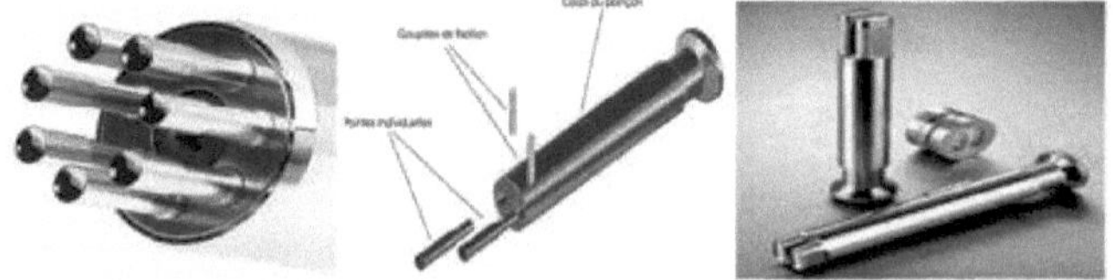

Figure 51: Examples of multi-point and micro-point fistons (111)

3.1.12- Condition of the turret and dies

It is extremely important to ensure that the equipment is adequately lubricated during each installation, even if an automatic lubrication system is used. Automated lubrication systems generally require approximately 10 to 15 minutes of continuous operation before the lubricating oil reaches the knobs and cams. During this phase, the effects of frictional wear and heating phenomena can increase considerably, leading to reduced play in the follower guides, increased wear on the cams and heads, and finally, the risk of the turret jamming.

The need for lubrication remains just as relevant when it comes to the prolonged storage of a tablet press or removable turret. Environmental conditions, in terms of temperature and humidity, can lead to the rapid spread of corrosion. In addition, used die housings are also the source of corroded dies (fretting), identifiable by the appearance of rust spots around the outside diameter of the upper part of the dies (Figures 52 and 53). In this context, simply replacing the dies will not resolve the issue in question. Similarly, adding a wear plate to restore a smooth surface in the die chamber is not a sustainable solution. Because the die housing is always oversized, the die retains a margin of movement in its housing, encouraging fretting and further deterioration of the die.

In addition, when the die set screws are tightened, they tend to move out of alignment with the punch guides, creating the potential for punch tip damage, punch head and cam wear, and excessive ejection forces (112).

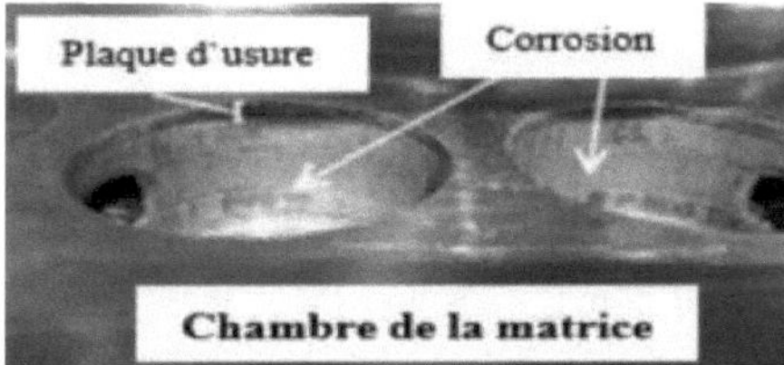

Figure 52: Illustration of corrosion in the die chambers (112)

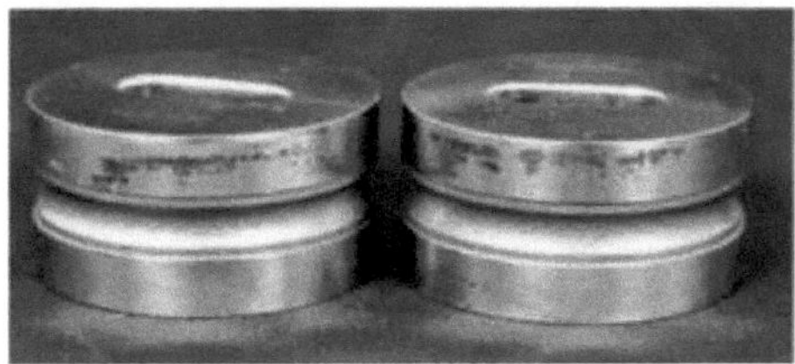

Figure 53: Die corrosion (112)

3.1.13- Polishing

In addition to coatings as a strategy for minimising or resolving adhesion and/or abrasion problems, tip polishing represents an alternative that can avoid many adhesion problems without resorting to costly solutions such as those involving coatings. The various advantages conferred by tip polishing can be summarised as follows:

• Maintaining the quality of compression surfaces, including tips.

• Improving the roughness of compression surfaces, helping to minimise and/or eliminate adhesion tendencies.

• Reduced mechanical friction during the compression process, resulting in improved machine life.

• Making format cleaning easier and more efficient. (74)

In the pharmaceutical sector, various strategies are used to monitor the condition of punches and dies. However, there is a misconception that suggests that once the first dimensional check is carried out on receipt of the punches, no further checks are required, and that punches are only replaced when they no longer meet the quality requirements of the tablet. Today, however, pharmaceutical companies are tending to adopt a policy of in-process control. This policy allows early detection of worn tooling, enabling it to be replaced or updated before the quality of the final product is compromised (74).

As a general rule, polishing should only be undertaken when powder residues remain on the tips, even after cleaning with isopropyl alcohol. However, some powder mixtures can be very abrasive and may damage the coating itself. In such situations, polishing may be necessary after each batch in order to preserve the quality of the tip and prevent further deterioration.

However, it should be noted that polishing must be carried out with appropriate brushes and pastes, such as diamond paste for example, and with extreme caution to avoid any risk of further damage to the tip (113).

Incorrect polishing could cause damage to the point, such as rounding of the external diameter, angles, engravings or even deformation of the concavity.

In industries where abrasive formulas are used all the time, the purchase of an automatic polisher could be a wise investment.

4- Operating parameters

The development of a pharmaceutical compression process involves the manipulation of a number of operating parameters to ensure the quality, reproducibility and efficiency of the process. For each product, the compression operating parameters are defined in advance so that the operator can follow these instructions and obtain tablets to the required specifications. These parameters are defined using the following methods:

4.1- Determining the overfill cam

The design of the cam will be determined on the basis of the usual properties of the granule, taking its bulk volume as a starting point, and using the following formulae (54):

Firstly, based on particle size analysis, it is essential to obtain the bulk density of the mixture using the following relationship:

$$\text{Density} = \frac{Masse\ testée}{Volume}$$

with mass in grams and volume in millilitres.

Next, we determine the volume of powder corresponding to the mass of a tablet:

$$\text{Volume} = \frac{Masse\ du\ comprimé}{Densité}$$

If the mass is in milligrams, the volume will be in mm^3 .

Finally, we will calculate the height of the powder corresponding to the volume using the dimensions of the tablets in millimetres, neglecting the volume corresponding to the arrow of the tablet in this consideration.

For round tablets, the diameter of the tablet is used:

$$\text{Height} = \frac{4x Volume}{\pi\ x\ Diametre^2}$$

For rectangular or square tablets:

$$\text{Height} = \frac{Volume}{Longueur\ x\ Largeur}$$

For oblong or oval compresses: use the previous equation, assuming that the cross-section of the compress can be assimilated to a rectangle for calculation purposes.

For triangular tablets :

$$\text{Height} = 2\ x\ \frac{Volume}{Base\ x\ Hauteur}$$

The cam to be used for the first tests will be twice the calculated value, rounded up to the nearest higher value. To illustrate, if the calculated height is 5.6 mm, a 12 mm cam will be used (54).

4.2- Determining machine speed

The optimum press speed will be determined by the ability to minimise the variation in filling with the selected overfill cam. Depending on the type of tablet press, this

filling variation is presented in a variety of ways, and acceptance criteria vary (generally between 7 and 10% for force-regulated presses, and less than 1% for displacement-regulated presses):

If, with the cam chosen, it is impossible to achieve a value below the target, the higher overfill cam will be chosen, or the rate will be reduced. All subsequent tests must be carried out at the rate thus determined. If, during qualification, it is necessary to change this rate, the tests already carried out must be repeated at the new rate (114).

4.3- Determining the precompression/compression torque

When the tablet press is equipped with two ramps (double output), the tests below can be carried out on a single ramp, and the precompression value chosen subsequently can be checked on the second ramp (81):

Initially, it is necessary to check that the mass of the tablets conforms to the specifications and is close to the target. Next, it is necessary to vary the pre-compression force and the compression force in order to scan the possible range of pre-compression/compression combinations. A minimum of 4 different pre-compression forces and 5 different compression forces per pre-compression force is recommended.

For each precompression/compression pair, the hardness, its coefficient of variation (CV) and the thickness are measured over 10 tablets. From these results, it is possible to plot a curve of hardness versus compression force for each pre-compression force, as well as a graph of the CV of the hardnesses for each pre-compression force.

These graphs will be used to determine the best pre-compression force/compression force ratio. The values selected must lie in the linear part of the hardness curve, before the plateau (values from which the hardness no longer increases with increasing compression force), in order to obtain the hardness value closest to the target (generally the median value of the product hardness specification included in the batch file).

Ideally, the ratio of pre-compression force to compression force should remain below 40%. If this is not the case, attempts can be made to reduce the compression rate. If the press is equipped with two ramps, it is useful to plot the hardness against the compression force, for verification purposes, on the second ramp of the machine, at the pre-compression value determined on the first ramp.

In this case, the test will be considered compliant if the curves of the two ramps are superimposable (54).

4.4- Determining the optimum penetration of the top fist at precompression and compression

The aim of this calculation is to check whether the penetration height of the upper fist allows identical kinematics between the upper and lower fist. If this is not the case, the distribution of forces inside the tablet is not symmetrical, which can result in cleavage or sticking, particularly with sensitive products. Symmetrical adjustment also enables the work to be distributed evenly between the upper and lower punches, thus reducing wear.

The machine must be set up in accordance with the target masses and hardnesses. To calculate the theoretical penetration of the fist at precompression, the following equation (54) is used:

$$\text{Pre-compression fist penetration} = \frac{h - EP}{2}$$

With h being the filling height and EP representing the air gap at precompression (The air gap being the distance between the top and bottom pumps at the time of precompression).

Then, for compression, we use the following equation:

$$\text{Penetration of the pompom on compression} = \frac{e - EC}{2}$$

With e corresponding to the thickness of the pre-compression and EC to the compression gap.

In order to check these heights, the penetrations calculated previously are applied, then the compression curve is determined again at the optimum precompression determined. If there is an improvement in the ease with which hardness can be obtained or an expansion of the usable range, this adjustment will be valid. If this is not the case, the initial setting for the penetration of the upper point is restored (54).

4.5- Determining the optimum spool valve speed

The test is conducted using the machine's standard distributor. Once the machine is set up with the target mass and target forces, the procedure is as follows:

The speed of the spool valve(s) is varied between the minimum and maximum values. For each machine ramp and each spool valve speed :

- Weigh 20 tablets, and adjust each point if necessary.
- The compression force and its coefficient of variation are recorded
- A UDM (Uniformity of Dosage Units) test is then carried out, and the coefficient of variation associated with this test is noted.

The optimum value for the valve speed represents a compromise between the variation in compression force and the value of the coefficient of variation of the UDM (115).

4.6- Determining tolerance and hysteresis

4.6.1- Theoretical principles and regulatory requirements

As far as tolerance is concerned, the limits we set will be those defined by pharmacopeia (mass uniformity). As for hysteresis, this will depend on the average mass limits that the laboratory wishes to maintain. In fact, no specific details are given on this subject in the regulatory texts (81).

The underlying principle is that if a process is sufficiently capable of maintaining the proposed mass deviations, the probability of finding T1s (T1 being the limit deviation as a percentage of the average mass) in conforming production will itself be very low. In a way, this is a statistical process control approach. However, technological advances now make it possible to guarantee the total absence of T1 in production.

The tolerance is calculated so that the press ejects the tablet as soon as its weight reaches that of a T1.

With regard to the above-mentioned mass uniformity test, pharmacopeia recommends weighing 20 tablets taken at random and calculating the average mass. The sample passes the test if the individual mass of no more than 2 of the 20 units deviates from the average mass by more than the percentage shown in the table (table 2), and if the mass of no unit deviates by more than twice this percentage (T2).

The aim of the linearity curve is to calculate the parameters that enable the press to maintain the recommended average mass limits, while ejecting any T1/T2 in order to avoid their presence in compliant production (54).

4.6.2- Determining tolerances

The purpose of this step is to check the linearity of the mathematical function: Compressive force = f(Mass).

From this relationship, the aim is to calculate the press tolerances, i.e. to determine the force values from which the press will eject the comprimes produced. Calculating the press tolerances involves determining the force values corresponding to tolerances T1 and T2.

The equation: Compressive force = f (Mass) to a straight line of the type Y = ax + b will be considered acceptable if the coefficient of determination R^2 of this relationship is greater than or equal to 0.97.

Measures to be implemented (54):

The machine must be warm (to prevent disturbances caused by the expansion of the fistons), and the weight must be set to the target.

The limits of the tolerance study must be at least (Target- T1) to (Target+T1), and ideally, (Target-T2) and (Target+T2) if these settings can be physically obtained. In fact, depending on the products and machines, the -T2 and +T2 values may not be achieved: too little mass may mean that the tablets are not hard enough to handle and, conversely, too much mass may mean that the compression force exceeds the overload limit of the fistons.

The test consists of recording force values for mass settings distributed as evenly as possible between the minimum and maximum bounds. The tests start with the lowest force value and progress towards the highest force value, without going backwards. It is imperative to allow the machine to stabilise for at least 3 minutes before taking the corresponding tablets for each measurement (based on the percentage change in compression force displayed on the control screen).

The number of measurements made is not restricted, but rather determined by the compression range. The masses, far from necessarily being rounded values, are methodically distributed between the two extremes of the study, approximately balancing the number of values both below the low boundary and the target, and between the target and the high boundary. A set of 13 values is considered optimal, while a number below 7 is considered insufficient. If possible, it is advisable to carry out a test close to "sensitive" values such as -T2, -T1, Target, +T1 and +T2.

Note: If the coefficient of determination is less than 0.97, it is imperative to check the calibration and correct mechanical operation of the press sensors. If there is no improvement, the limits of the study can be reduced from T2 to T1. If the coefficient remains below 0.97, the press cannot be qualified as it stands. To remedy this situation, improvements should be sought in the following areas:

- Cold machine: For optimum determination of tolerances, the machine must be hot. Otherwise, the test could be falsified by variations in the length of the pins.

- Inadequate compression force: Compression must not be carried out in the linear part of the force-hardness relationship

- Problems with the press itself: compensator spheres, various clearances, tool wear

- Compression range inadequate

Once the coefficients have been obtained, the forces corresponding to the target mass and to masses -T1 and +T1 can be calculated using the equation "Compression force = f(Mass)":

- Force (Target) = a x Mass (Target) + b
- Force (-T1) = a X mass (-T1) + b
- Force (+T1) = a x Mass (+T1) + b

We can then determine the tolerance defined as follows:

$$\text{Tolerance (Calculated force)} = \frac{Force\ (+T_1) - Force\ (Cible)}{Force\ (Cible)} \times 100$$

To the force tolerance calculated by the above equation, a restrictive margin of 5% must be subtracted, corresponding to the maximum tolerated deviation in strain gauge accuracy (54).

4.6.3- Optimising regulation, determining hysteresis

The determination of the droop of the regulator (corresponding to the zone of non-regulation of the "mass" or "hysteresis") will be carried out using the equations and values obtained in the previous paragraph. The hysteresis will be evaluated at half the press adjustment limit.

Table 6: Adjustment and hysteresis limits as a function of compressor mass (54)

Compressed mass	Adjustment limit (%)	Hysteresis (%)
< 80 mg	± 1,9	± 0,95
> 80 and < 250 mg	± 1,4	± 0,70
> 250 mg	± 0,9	± 0,45

In the same way as the tolerance calculations mentioned above, it is possible to determine, using the compression masses associated with the upper and lower hysteresis limits, the forces corresponding to these masses. This gives the hysteresis of the compression force as a percentage (54).

4.6.4- Calculation of the adjustment parameter for roller spacing as a function of knuckle expansion

To calculate the value of this parameter, it is necessary to carry out the procedure cold after a pause of at least 8 hours (the time required for the press to cool down completely).

The first step is to set the press to the target mass, then record the compression and slice height values. The press should then be run for 3 hours in primary control mode. After this period, it is necessary to correct the mass, if necessary, in order to find exactly the initial mass.

Finally, the compression slice height is adjusted to exactly match the initial target force, and the new compression slice height (81) is noted.

4.6.5- Verification of pitch and respect for hysteresis

Pitch, defined as the amplitude by which the press adjusts the metering cam at each control in the primary control loop, is a vital measure for guaranteeing press reactivity in the event of a drift. To check whether this adjustable amplitude allows the press to return quickly to its hysteresis in the event of a deviation, the press can be set up with all the target values obtained (valve speeds, precompression, compression, tolerances and hysteresis), then switched to primary control mode.

The press is then left to run for two minutes to stabilise and the mass (the average mass over 20 tablets) is checked. Mass values corresponding to Mass (Target) ± (2 x Hysteresis) are then calculated, followed by Mass (Target) ± (3 x Hysteresis). We return to manual mode to vary the mass according to the values determined above, before returning to primary control. The mass is then checked after regulation, taking care to check the number of corrections made and the maximum return time.

The mass after regulation must be within the hysteresis, but need not be equal to the starting mass (54).

4.7- Dwell time calculation and determination

Dwell time is defined as the part of the contact time during which the points do not change their vertical position in relation to the rollers, i.e. when the flat part of the point head is in contact with the rollers. Note that the Dwell tim does not depend on the diameter of the roller.

The notion of Dwell time is widely misused or misunderstood. In fact, it should be used as a reference, a measure of linear velocity (i.e. tangential or angular) and therefore depends on the geometry of the point's head. Velocity comparisons based on Dwell time assume that the point has a flat head. The speed is then the length of this flat portion divided by the dwell time. For the same line speed, the smaller the flat head of the dot, the shorter the Dwell time. The compression time for dome-shaped punch heads is virtually zero by definition, regardless of the line speed of the press. This is why, compared with compression time, line speed is a better measure of press speed.

Any attempt to calculate Dwell time from compression time traces is doomed to failure because such a curve depends on the properties of the compressed powder material. Plastic deformation and elastic recovery distort the 'ideal' shape of the force-time profile.

A simple "classic" formula for stopping time does not take into account the curvature of the trajectory

DT(ms) = (L x NS x 3600,000) / (n x PCD x TPH)

Or L = Length of a flat portion of the fist (mm)

NS = Number of stations

n = 3.14159265

PCD = Turret pitch circle diameter (mm)

TPH = Press speed in terms of tablets per hour

In fact, the Dwell time as defined depends on the geometry of the tooling. A linear (tangential) turret speed is a better way of representing the press speed independently of the geometry of the punch head (81).

5- Conclusion

Compression is a complex process to develop because of the variability of the materials to be compressed and the properties of these raw materials. This presentation enabled us to take an in-depth look at the mechanisms involved in compression. Equipment has evolved in line with the understanding of these mechanisms, and each piece of equipment has its own specific features that need to be taken into account.

Therefore, knowledge of all the parameters influencing the final quality of the compressed product is essential. We have seen that taking all these variables into account enables the developer and then the manufacturer to successfully complete projects, whatever the material to be compressed. Research into the fine-tuning of these parameters is carried out throughout the process, during the research and development phase of the formula, the development of the process as well as during its fine-tuning when a new press is acquired. However, all these parameters are more or less interdependent, and developers or manufacturers have to make choices and compromises to give priority to certain properties and according to the different constraints. Development is generally carried out empirically, but knowledge of the parameters and their impact can save time by guiding choices and anticipating the consequences.

Although the process seems to be well mastered nowadays, manufacturing faults frequently occur for which manufacturers still do not seem to have found a radical solution, resulting in considerable losses when they occur. The fourth and final chapter will be devoted to the study of the mechanisms of occurrence of the various interactions with the tooling and to the optimisation of the process based on recent research data aimed at finding solutions to these problems, improving the performance of the presses, as well as other possibilities for increasing yield. Process monitoring is also being developed to improve robustness and reproducibility, with research focusing on the possibility of monitoring production in real time in order to react in the event of parameter deviations, and to enable the process to be fully automated as a future prospect.

INTERACTIONS WITH TOOLING AND POINTS FOR OPTIMISING THE COMPRESSION PROCESS

1- Interaction with tooling and compression faults

Compression can be defective at different levels:

• Deficiency in terms of hardness, necessitating a re-evaluation of the parameters of the compression process, with an increase in the compression force, combined with a reformulation of the blend, which has proved unsuitable for the manufacture of tablets.

• The uniformity problem suggests variations in process parameters over time and/or non-uniformity of the initial mix, including segregation phenomena during storage or feeding.

• Defective tablets, where the nature of the defect generally gives an indication of the underlying cause of the problem (116)

Questioning can involve the formulation as well as the operating conditions (process parameters) and the equipment. The origins of the manufacturing defect can therefore be multiple, and the use of an ISHIKAWA diagram, also known as a fishbone diagram, can be beneficial in identifying the origin of the problem (117).

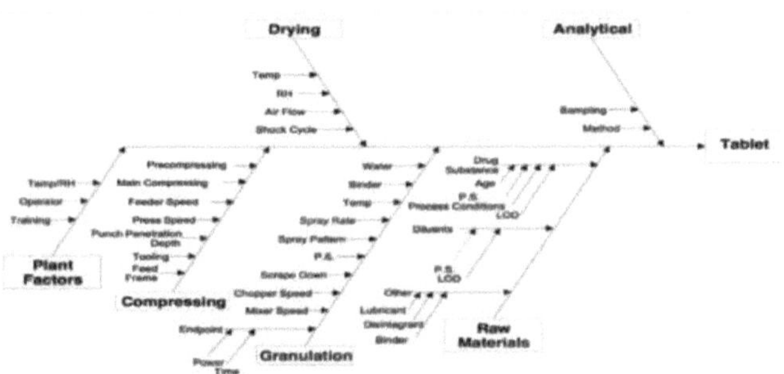

Figure 54: Ishikawa diagram of the possible causes of the various faults

of tablets (117)

Among the most common and documented faults occurring during compression are :

1.1- Bare, patented tablets

At the end of the press or during the handling operations following compression, it is not uncommon to find broken tablets. This defect is manifested by a break in the edges of the tablet and is generally attributable to inappropriate settings on the tablet press.

More specifically, it is essential to check the adjustment of the ejection ramp and to ensure that the trajectory of the tablets in the transfer ramp to the dust collector remains orderly. If this is not the case, the tablets may collide, increasing the risk of fragmentation (109,110).

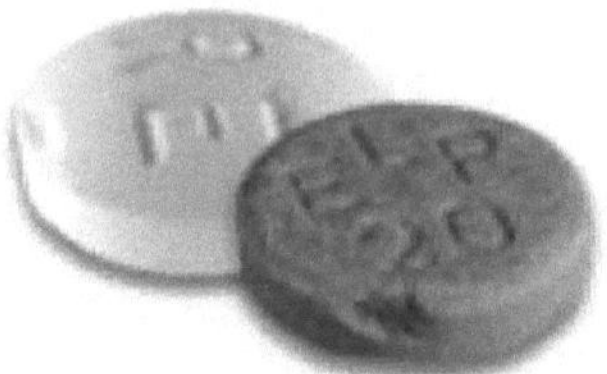

Figure 55: Example of an ebreche tablet (119)

1.2- Bare cracked tablets

Cracks, or small breaks, refer to compresses that show cracks on their upper and lower central surfaces, and sometimes even on their sides. These cracks may be the result of excessively rapid elastic recovery of the tablet after compression. Similarly, the use of fistons with a pronounced concavity is an additional factor conducive to the appearance of this phenomenon (118).

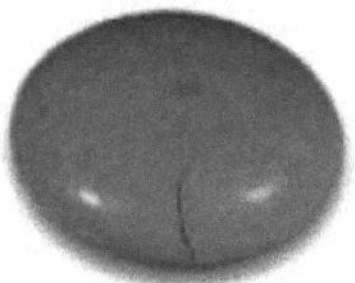

Figure 56: Example of a cracked tablet (119)

1.3- Plain flu tablets

The term tablet seizure in the die refers to the situation where tablets adhere to or break off inside the die. In effect, a film forms in the die, hindering the tablet ejection process. In the event of excessive adhesion, cracks may appear on the sides of the tablet, eventually leading to its crumbling.

The most common causes of this problem are excessive moisture in the grain, insufficient lubrication of the outer phase, and/or the use of worn matrices (74).

1.4- Bare tablets with black dots on the surface

The term "blackheads" covers a range of defects related to the visual appearance of tablets, which may take the form of spots rather than simple dots, be grey rather than black, or even appear as spots inside the tablet rather than on its surface.

There are many possible causes for these spots or blackheads. However, if these imperfections appear on the surface of the tablet and do not seem to be integrated into the core of the tablet, it is very likely that the press is the cause rather than the powder mix.

As the compression cycles progress, the abrasive action of the powders causes some parts of the equipment to erode. It is not the equipment itself that is responsible for the black spots (unless poor quality material is used), but rather the consequence of wear on the pins and dies, increasing the initial clearance that allowed them to slide. The extra space can then trap particles in the mix. When these particles accumulate on the wall of the die, the friction from passing the punch can burn this material, depositing black particles on the surface of the compacts during compression. Aggressive cleaning and excessive polishing of the equipment can encourage or accelerate the appearance of such defects. Rounding the angle of the edge of the fist head can also allow particles to become trapped between the fist and the die, creating black spots. So, when black spots appear during compression, the first check to be made concerns the condition of the punches and dies (109,110).

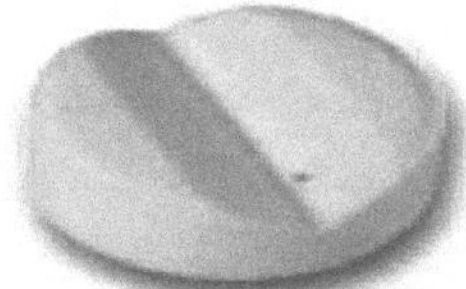

Figure 57: Example of a tablet with black dots (119)

1.5- Collage

The phenomenon of bonding refers to the adhesion of powders to the surfaces of compression tools, i.e. the upper and lower punches and the walls of the die. In the literature, several definitions of this phenomenon exist due to its different variants. Briefly, there are three main types of bonding: "Picking", where the powder adheres to the grooves engraved on the surface of the fistons; "Filming", where the face of the fistons is covered by a film of powder; and "Sticking", where the surfaces of the fistons or dies are covered by several layers of powder(96,97). The term 'sticking' is therefore used to group together all these phenomena into a single term.

Sticking rarely occurs during the formulation development phase, when only a few tablets are produced. It generally appears during the large-scale production phases, where the possibilities for modification and investigation are very limited. At this scale, gluing causes serious damage to production: it increases costs and production times, affects the quality of the tablets produced and causes premature wear of presses and tools.

When sticking occurs, production is interrupted to clean, polish and/or replace the punches before resuming. The tablets then have a deteriorated appearance, with rough surfaces, incomplete engraving and variations in weight, leading to their rejection and destruction(96,98). The occurrence of bonding can also lead to premature wear of the fistons due to the high ejection forces. Despite the considerable progress made, no fundamental cause has yet been identified to fully understand the phenomenon of bonding. This is due to its complex multifactorial nature and the long unavailability of appropriate evaluation techniques to measure it (96,98,99,100).

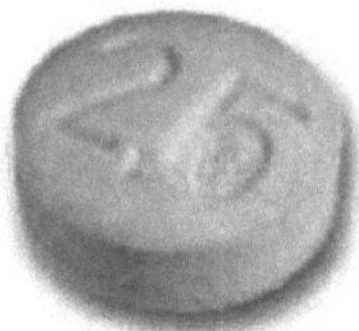

Figure 58: Example of a tablet that has been fist-bonded (119)

1.5.1- Bonding mechanisms

1.5.1.1- Sticking due to air trapping

During the compression process, particularly when using concave fists, a variable volume of air is trapped in the fist cup. The increased depth of this cup increases the propensity to trap air. This air trapping creates an area of low density on the top of the tablet, and when the top fist rises after compression, some of the grain can adhere to its surface.

To overcome this problem, it is essential to ensure that the dwell time of the punch is correctly set to optimise the evacuation of air from the powder mixture in the die. More pre-compression also allows more air to be removed before the compression stage, reducing the volume of air that can be trapped.

The height of compression in the die is also a crucial parameter. By adjusting the penetration depth of the top die into the die to the optimum level, air can escape easily and quickly during compression. Where it is not possible to adjust these parameters, an alternative is to use tapered dies, thus facilitating air evacuation during compression (125).

1.5.1.2- Sticking due to a lubrication problem

The inherent function of a lubricant in the formulation of a product lies in its ability to prevent adhesion of the powder to punches, dies and other components of the tablet press. In addition, the lubricant used in the formulation facilitates the ejection of compacted tablets.

These substances, magnesium stearate being the most commonly used, are characterised by a fine particle size and are present in very low proportions in the mix. However, the lubricant has a significant influence on the ability to produce quality tablets. In the absence of adequate mixing after incorporation, particularly in the case of non-homogeneous mixing, their effectiveness will not be optimal. Two errors frequently encountered when applying lubricants are as follows:

•   The first is to neglect the preliminary sieving of lubricants in order to eliminate granular and oversized particles.

•   The second is the failure to mix the lubricant evenly in the product formula. During the compression process, the absence of lubricant in the mix may cause squeaking within the press. The ejection force will also be significantly higher than the norm, which could lead to damage to the punches and cams. In the absence or inadequate mixing of the lubricant, gluing problems may also occur. The most common misdiagnosis when such a gluing problem occurs is to focus exclusively on the tooling. In fact, once the sticking has been detected, the most common action taken by compression operators is to stop the press, remove the sticky product and polish the punches before restarting production. Although this action temporarily solves the sticking problem, it leads to a false conclusion as to the origin of the problem. The sticking would reappear, forcing the press to stop during production and the need to polish the punches again. Thus, at the end of the batch, the loss of polishing of the tooling is often wrongly identified as the source of the problem (125).

1.5.1.3- Sticking due to poor control of grain drying

During a poorly controlled drying process, a problem of surface hardening of the grains can emerge, manifested by granules that dry on the surface while remaining damp on the inside. This can occur when the binder is not evenly distributed in the mix and drying is incomplete. However, it can also occur when the binder is correctly added, but the drying process of the grain is too rapid.

In this situation, the rapid elimination of the intrinsic water causes part of the binder to move to the outside of the granule. This leads to drying and the formation of a hard layer around the rest of the material, which can no longer dry evenly. In such circumstances, the sticking phenomenon can be caused by two distinct aspects: residual moisture in the centre of the granule and excess binder concentrated on the surface of the granule.

The recommended solution to this problem is to slow down the drying process. In a persistent situation where the product presents bonding problems despite a methodical diagnosis, the use of a coating on the knuckles can be considered. As mentioned above, a chromium nitride (CrN) coating will, among other things, improve resistance to adhesion problems. In some cases, this measure may be enough to put an end to the bonding problem. However, it is important to note that modifying the tooling can also be a waste of time and money, as many products can exhibit bonding problems regardless of modifications to the fist design (125).

1.5.1.4- Target collage on fist motifs

Another problem frequently encountered during production is the sticking together of material concentrated in the knuckle patterns, also known as "picking". This term is used when only a small amount of material in a tablet has a sticking problem.

This problem generally occurs on the top fistons and worsens during the process as more and more material adheres to the material already present. Picking thus represents a particular type of gluing where the particles of the grain adhere to the letters, logos and other patterns on the face of the knuckle. In general, the glued material is found at the level of the numbers and letters known as 'closed', forming 'islands'. These numbers include 0, 4, 6, 8 and 9. Similarly, the letters most affected by picking are A/a, B/b, D/d, e, P/p, Q/q (125).

The figure below shows a round tablet with the number "9". To reduce or eliminate picking problems concentrated in the central island of the "9", it is possible to incorporate a pre-embossing feature into the design of the tooling. This feature implies that the face of the punch comprises an island which is not as deep as the rest of the embossing (126).

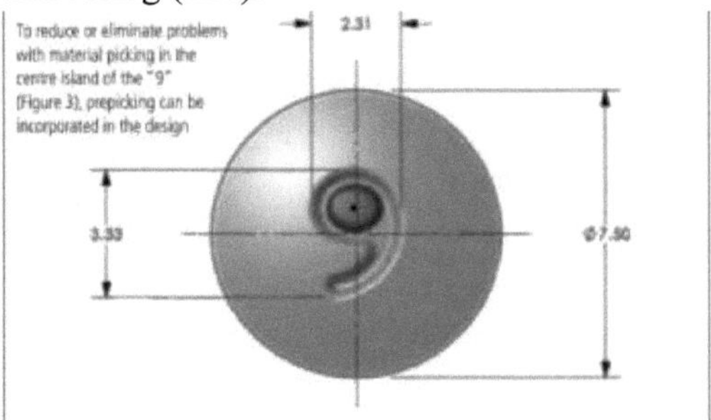

Figure 59: Schematic representation of an engraving of the number "9" on a round tablet (126)

The figure below shows an example of an island where the depth is reduced by 50% (from 0.33 mm to 0.17 mm). This reduction in depth can vary from 10 to 100%, depending on the extent of the bonding problem. However, when such a modification is made, it is crucial to ensure that the engraving remains legible, particularly if the process includes a tablet coating step (126).

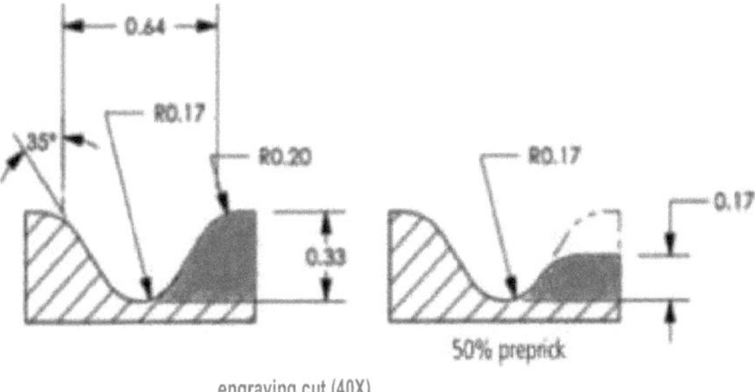

Figure 60: Schematisation of a peripiquage on a "9" engraving

(126)
1.6- The divide
According to many authors, the term 'cleavage' is a concept that encompasses two possible defects that can occur during compression: lamination and debonding. The main cause generally put forward is the presence of air trapped and compressed with the material. Air, being easily compressible, has elastic properties. Therefore, after compression, it expands within the compressed mass, causing separation. One of the most common solutions to this problem is to revise the pre-compression process to improve air removal prior to compression (127).

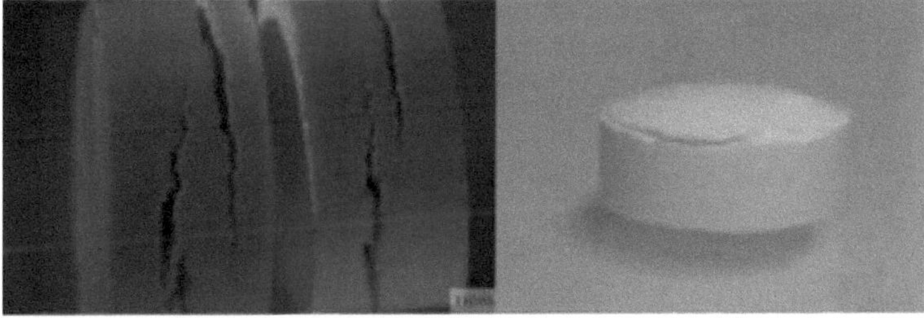
Figure 61: Clive compression (128)

However, many other phenomena can contribute to the appearance of cleavage. They will be presented here in order to understand their mechanisms and origins, so as to better identify and resolve them when they occur in production.
1.6.1- Capping or decapping
The cap, also known as the calotte, refers to the upper or lower part of a tablet that separates horizontally, partially or completely, from the main body of the tablet. This cap is generally detached when the tablet is ejected from the tablet press, but can also occur during subsequent handling. The phenomenon of capping or uncapping is generally due to the presence of air trapped inside the tablet during compression, and to the subsequent expansion of the tablet when it is ejected from the die.

The debulking problem can also result from too low a residual moisture content after wet granulation (grain too dry). In this case, it will be necessary to adjust the moisture content during the wetting stage and optimise the specifications for the drying stage.

In addition, debonding can be caused by using too weak a binder, although this does not apply to mass production, but rather to the development stage. In this situation, it will be necessary to use a more effective binder.

Lastly, poor tool maintenance can be the cause of debottlenecking. Poorly polished or worn fists and dies will encourage this problem. For example, the presence of J-shaped hooks, a distinctive wear pattern, at the lower end of the fist. In fact, as the surface wears, a J-shaped hook can become transformed at the end of the fist, exacerbating, in particular, the defects of the uncapping (118).

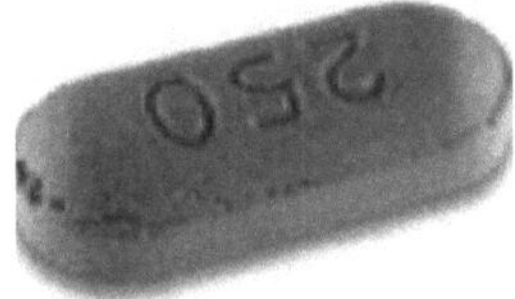

Figure 62: Example of a tablet that has been debottlenecked (119)

1.6.2- Lamination

Laminating, also known as lamination, refers to the separation of a film into two or more distinct horizontal layers. Unlike debottlenecking, where only the cap separates from the rest of the tablet, lamination involves dividing the body of the tablet itself into two or more layers. This type of rupture is favoured by the low thickness of the tablet combined with high compression pressure (129).

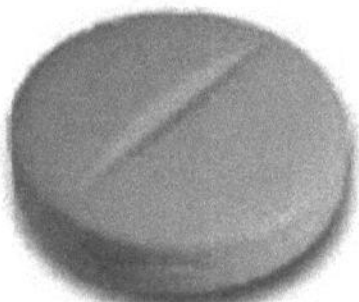

Figure 63: Example of a tablet that has undergone the rolling process (119)

1.6.2.1- Understanding debottlenecking and rolling mechanisms

Thanks to the work of Vincent Mazel in his study entitled "Etude de la compression pharmaceutique a l'aide d'une approche de mecanique des milieux continus" (130), we will be looking at the physical mechanisms behind the phenomena of debottlenecking and lamination. This more technical approach will enable us to gain an in-depth understanding of these mechanisms, thus facilitating the identification of the real causes of these defects during production and paving the way for their resolution. The various aspects discussed will be based on the study of biconvex tablets, the latter being the most frequently encountered in pharmaceutical production.

1.6.2.2-Density distribution in biconvex tablets

A comparison of the density distribution between a flat tablet and a biconvex tablet reveals a significant difference. The biconvex tablet has a significantly less dense zone towards the centre, with a more heterogeneous overall distribution.

To understand this phenomenon, we need to look at relative deformation. During compression, the two punches (upper and lower) come into motion, and all the points on the surface of their cups experience the same displacement. However, the distance between the edges of these cups will be less than the distance between their centres.

Since relative deformation is the ratio of displacement to initial distance, it will be more pronounced at the edges of the point than at the centre of the cup. It is therefore logical, as shown in Figure 64, to see an area of high density at the edges of the compact and a lower density at the centre (130).

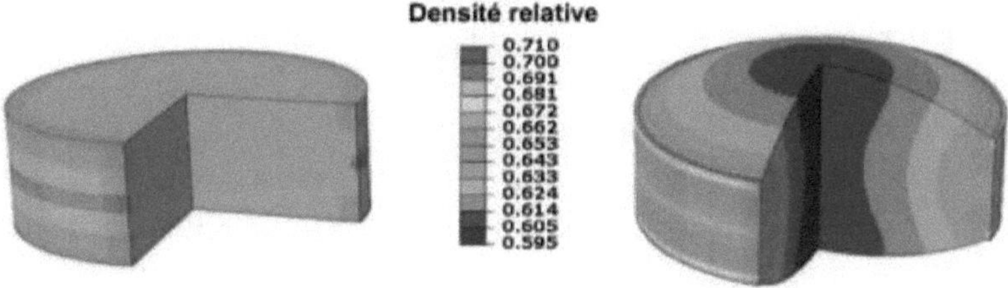

Figure 64: Comparison of the distribution between a flat tablet and a biconvex tablet (130)

Two crucial parameters need to be analysed in depth when studying the density distribution: the curvature of the fist and the thickness of the tablet.

1.6.1.3- Fist curvature

In the figure below, it can be seen that the area of least compression density is in the centre of the cup. In addition, as the punch has a more pronounced curvature, i.e. a smaller radius of curvature, this area becomes less dense (130).

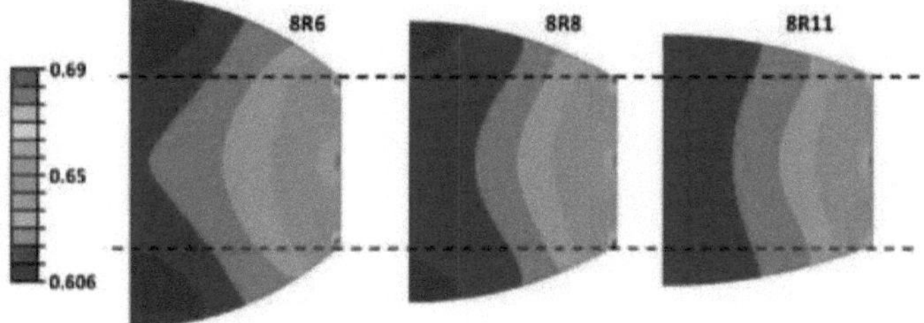

Figure 65: Distribution of density as a function of fist curvature (130)

1.6.1.4- Influence of thickness

The force exerted on the powder mixture is divided into two distinct components, as illustrated in Figure 66: the axial pressure, aligned in the same direction as the axis of the fistons, and the radial pressure, perpendicular to the first.

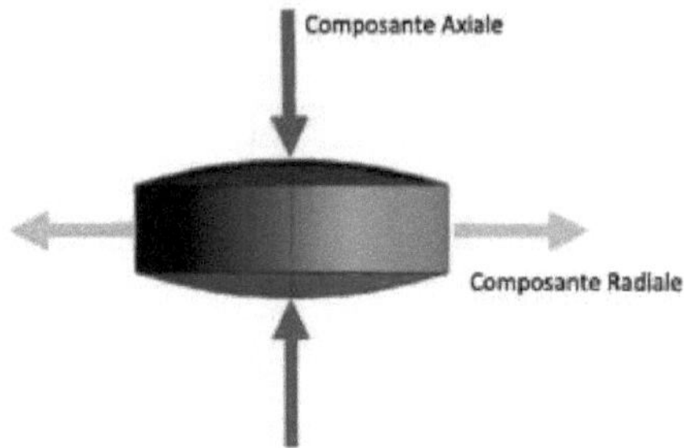

Figure 66: Breakdown of the pressure applied to the compressor (130)

By analysing the variation in radial pressure as a function of axial pressure, significant distinctions were observed between flat and biconvex tablets, taking into account a key variable: thickness.

Flat tablets show a thickness-independent trend for both components (radial pressure and axial pressure). On the other hand, biconvex tablets show a variation in radial pressure as a function of thickness, inducing a variation in relative density.

The evolution of relative density as a function of thickness is as follows:

- Flat tablet :

• Little influence of thickness

• Increasing the thickness of the tablet will result in a slight overall decrease in relative density (due to increased friction in the matrix as a result of the thickness).

- Biconvex tablet :

• Significant influence of thickness

• As the thickness decreases, the relative density will decrease at the centre of the compact and increase at its edge.

This feature highlights the importance of controlling thickness during compression. In fact, a simple change in the thickness of a biconvex tablet is essentially equivalent to an adjustment in the compressive stresses applied to it. By controlling this parameter precisely, many quality problems can be avoided.

It is essential to note that even if two biconvex tablets of different thicknesses are produced in the same operation without changing the press pressure parameters, they will be considered as separate objects, with different mechanical properties (130).

1.6.1.5- Debottlenecking mechanisms

• Elastic recovery, radial pressure and shear stress

The elastic recovery undergone by the tablet after compression varies significantly depending on the profile of the tablet, whether it is flat or biconvex. In the case of a biconvex tablet, the specific nature of the elastic recovery is of particular importance, contributing to a better understanding of the debottlenecking phenomenon.

Once the powder mixture has been compressed, with the top fist reaching its maximum depth, it is relevant to compare the separation phase between the fist and the shaped tablet. A clear distinction then emerges between a flat tablet and a biconvex tablet:

• In the first case, contact between the fist and the compressor is broken almost simultaneously over the entire contact surface, at the moment when the axial pressure reaches zero.

• For biconvex fists, the loss of contact occurs progressively between the fist and the compress. It starts at the edge, then gradually spreads to the entire surface(130).

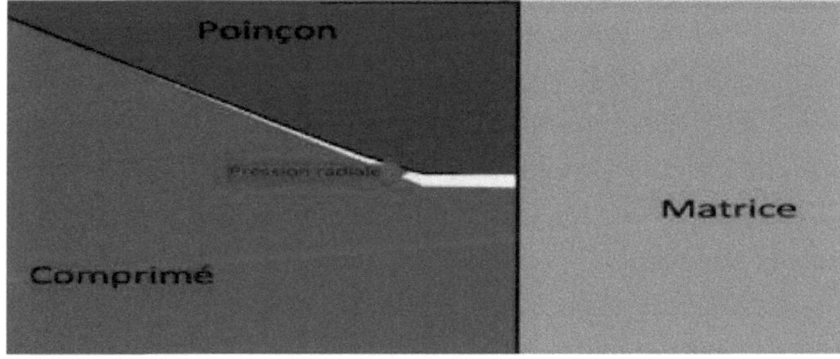

Figure 67: Illustration of the zone of loss of contact between the fist and the biconvex tablet (130)

The gradual progression of this loss of contact is not without consequences for the evolution of the radial pressure. In fact, a transient increase in this component is observed inside the compressor just before the axial pressure reaches zero.

This phenomenon is explained by the fact that the part corresponding to the edge of the tablet always remains laterally stressed by the matrix, while the cap of the tablet is stress-free. The result is an elastic overlap that is both axial and radial. The singularity of this overlap leads to the development of a shear stress (whose evolution is shown in the figure below) at the boundary between the cap and the 'pavement' of the tablet (the flat part between the cap and the edge). It is important to emphasise that it is precisely at this point that rupture occurs, corresponding to the phenomenon of debottlenecking of biconvex tablets (130).

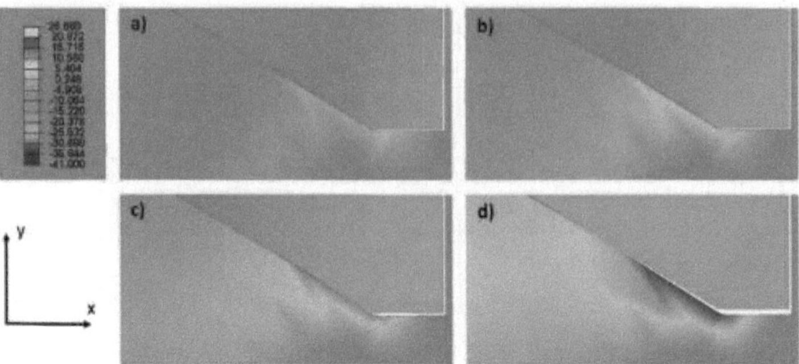

Figure 68: Evolution of shear stress at the end of decompression (130)

The particular phenomenon of the elastic covering of the biconvex tablet, which gives rise to a shear stress at the edge of the cap, seems likely to be responsible for its propensity to unseat. Consequently, in the production environment, it is imperative to take into consideration the fact that the use of a fist with a small radius of curvature (a large concavity) will accentuate the shear stress, thus increasing the risk of debottlenecking.

1.6.1.6- Influence of the ejection phase on the debottlenecking phenomenon

Following the explanation given above, it would be expected that the debottlenecking phenomenon would occur systematically on both sides of the tablet. However, asymmetrical debottlenecking problems are frequently encountered, where only the top cap, the first to be ejected from the die, separates from the body of the tablet.

One explanation for this asymmetry could lie in the influence of the ejection phase, which is fundamentally asymmetrical. As long as the force exerted by the lower fist remains lower than the ejection force, the central part of the tablet does not move. The movement of the lower fist therefore causes the compression spring to deform.

A study of the evolution of the shear stress in the tablet showed that when the lower fist rises, causing the tablet to deform, this shear stress increases on the upper face and decreases on the lower face. As a result, there is an increased risk of debonding on the upper face at the start of the ejection phase. This phenomenon explains the emergence of compacts with only a debottlenecking of the upper face (130).

The role of the ejection force on the debottlenecking phenomenon can be summarised as follows:

- The greater the force required to eject the tablet, the greater the deformation it undergoes, thus increasing the risk of the top surface debottlenecking.

• Any parameter that increases the ejection force increases the risk of unseating the tablet produced.

Examples of situations that can increase the ejection force include poor lubrication, high speed, and worn dies. If there is a debottlenecking problem in production, it is imperative to monitor and adjust all these parameters in an attempt to remedy this quality defect (130).

1.6.2.1- Rolling mechanism

In this context, the mechanism at the origin of the rupture of the compression implies a stress different from that of the shear. In fact, it is a tensile stress that induces the horizontal separation of the compress.

This tensile stress evolves as a function of the thickness of the compact. As shown in Figure 69, at constant pressure, the early onset of lamination is proportional to the reduction in the thickness of the compact.

compressed. This is all the more reason why a low thickness favours

the emergence of areas of low density in the centre of the compact.

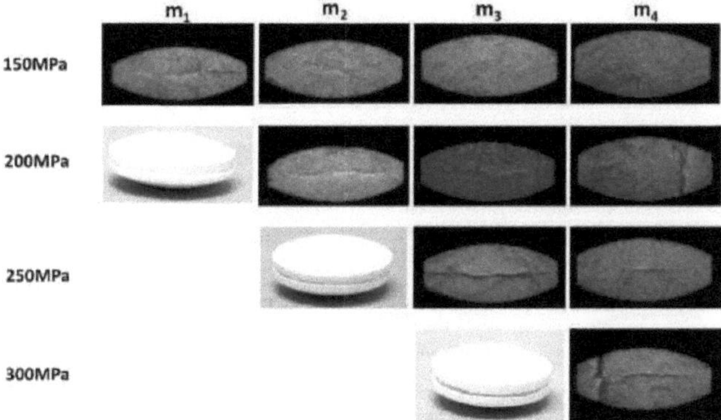

Figure 69: Impact of thickness on the rolling phenomenon (130)

These different images illustrate that the onset of compression fracture occurs at its centre. Depending on the compression parameters, the crack can then propagate to the edge, exposing the lamination phenomenon. This type of fracture is favoured by a low compression thickness and high compression pressure. Various tests have shown that the fracture of thicker compresses increases as the main compression pressure increases.

On the other hand, it is predictable that increasing the curvature of the compact will favour the emergence of cracks. Thus, rolling and debottlenecking share similar parameters that favour their occurrence. These two mechanisms are therefore in competition, and it is possible to observe the two phenomena simultaneously on compresses (130).

2- Optimising the compression process

2.1- Optimising the performance of tablet presses

In tablet production, regardless of batch size, a clear and consistent objective is to maximise the production of compliant tablets while minimising inevitable product losses. To increase throughput, tablet press manufacturers adjust various parameters such as the number of stations, turret speed, feed position, fill cam dimensions, tooling, blade position and reject parameters. This section will look at how to optimise the performance of a tablet press (131).

2.1.1- Increased turret speed

Where it is possible to increase press speed while maintaining acceptable levels of output, this is a first step towards optimising press efficiency. However, in the real world of pharmaceutical tablet production, most tablets are not made at maximum press speeds, as it is impossible to produce quality tablets at high speeds. Indeed, higher press speeds run the risk of inducing wide variability in tablet weight due to reduced die fill time, as well as lower tablet hardness due to a shorter compression time during which force is applied. Non-conforming compacts are rejected, impacting yields. It is therefore imperative to find a compromise between speed and yield (132).

2.1.2- Installation of interchangeable turrets

A second strategy for significantly increasing production performance is to use several turrets to maximise output for each tablet size. The turret is the central moving part of the tablet press, into which the punches are inserted.

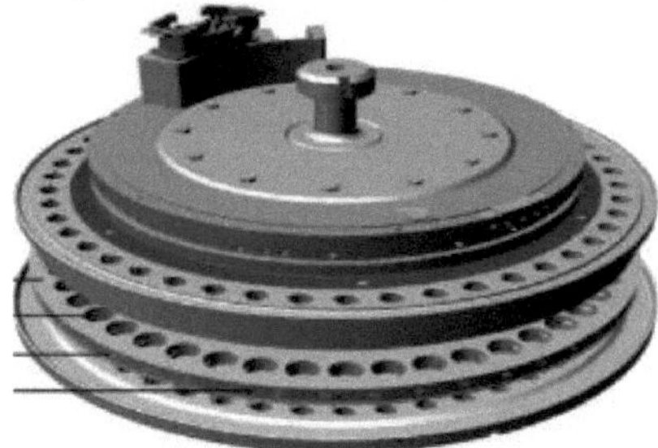

Figure 70: Diagram of a tablet press turret (35)

Most modern production machines offer a range of interchangeable turrets. By adjusting the tablet size to suit the turret selection, it is possible to maximise production across the entire product portfolio without the need to increase the validated speed range. In addition, the use of multiple turrets allows off-line preparation, cleaning and tooling, facilitating rapid changeover. This approach can have a significant impact on efficiency by significantly reducing overall downtime (132).

2.1.3- Reduced cleaning times

The previous point highlights the third option, which is to reduce cleaning times. To achieve this, the adoption of a standard changeover procedure, accompanied by a specially designed trolley to house the parts, can ensure a simplified and consistent method for assembling and disassembling the parts in a precise order, positioning them in a reproducible manner. To minimise overall changeover times, some companies opt to use a second set of parts, cleaned off-line and ready for use as soon as the previous batch has been completed.

As suggested earlier, the integration of an additional turret offers the opportunity to clean, prepare and tool turrets off-line, facilitating rapid changeover. By combining this additional turret strategy with a second set of parts and a streamlined changeover procedure, it is possible to reduce overall changeover time by up to 50% (133).

2.1.4- Automation strategy

The fourth option is based on automation strategies or transition to semi-supervised operation, where a single operator can monitor and operate several tablet presses simultaneously. This approach seems increasingly feasible given recent advances in modern tablet presses.

When it comes to feeding powder into the press, the operator positions a container over the press at the start of production, and the equipment is then automatically fed without any operator intervention required throughout the batch. This automation is common on most modern tablet presses.

The filling hoppers at the machine outlet must be changed periodically by the operator to enable the press to run continuously. However, most modern units combining dust extraction and metal control offer a lifting height and a tablet inverter that takes care of automatic feeding according to a predefined number of tablets. Depending on the size of the container, these systems can eliminate the need for the operator to handle the collection hoppers over an extended period of time, simply stopping the press once the last container has been filled, if the operator does not return in time.

The integration of an in-line tablet tester also enables tablet presses to be semi-automated. The tester measures the weight, thickness and hardness of individual compresses at predefined intervals and provides closed-loop feedback to the press force control system to keep the process focused on the compressed weight target. The main limitations of these systems are the capital investment required and the ability of automated testers to correctly align each tablet shape and size in a reproducible manner for consistent hardness measurement.

In general, a tablet compression system capable of handling tablet collection and periodic sampling with closed-loop feedback opens the door to semi-assisted operation, where a single operator can supervise and monitor the operation of several tablet presses simultaneously (133).

2.2- Current solutions to manufacturing defects

2.2.1- The divide

The data collected following a multivariate approach to cleavage (debottlenecking) highlighted the impact of the powder's rheological properties (pressure drop in the powder mixture, cohesion and air permeability) and mechanical properties (porosity, internal air pressure in the compact, etc.) on the occurrence of this phenomenon. The fact that the causes are so diverse means that the solutions can vary depending on the cause. To remedy the presence of air within low-density powders, it is possible to increase the density of the powder by wet granulation or compaction. Another solution is to reduce the speed of the press to allow better evacuation of the air trapped in the matrix (134).

The various solutions known to alleviate this problem of cleavage (decalottage), depending on the possible causes, are as follows:

Table 7: Possible causes of cleavage and solutions (74)

Possible causes	Possible solutions
Too many fine particles in the granule	Checking the particle size profile beforehand
Fragile and porous granules	Verification of the particle size profile Verification of the binding agent Verification of the process
The humidity of the pellets is too low	Check the drying process and residual humidity Add hygroscopic substances
Low proportion of binder or poor solubility of raw materials in the binder	Increase the quantity of binder Checking solubility
Insufficient or inadequate lubricant	Increase the quantity of lubricant Change lubricant
Poor quality punches	Pointer polishing Change of materials Change of supplier
Geometry of inadequate pins	Checking the design of the tablet
Incorrect adjustment of the lower punch displacement during rejection	Adjusting the configuration of machine parameters
Poorly lubricated punches or badly polished dies	Examination of the condition of punches and dies

The various solutions known to alleviate the problem of cracks, depending on the possible causes, are as follows:

Table 8: Possible causes of cracks and solutions (74)

Possible causes	Possible solutions
Low proportion of fines in the granule	Check the particle size profile Add fines
Excessively dry granules	Increasing the moisture content of the aggregate Add a binder or reduce the drying time
High concavity tool designs (Guns)	Checking tablet design Using special scrapers

2.2.3- Black spots

The various solutions known to alleviate the problem of cracks, depending on the possible causes, are as follows:

Table 9: Possible causes of cracks and solutions (74)

Possible causes	Possible solutions
Erode tools (abrasion, excessive polishing)	Inspection and renewal of tools
Damaged fist guide seal	New replacement
Scraper blade (wear, incorrect adjustment)	Replacement, adjustment
Excessive lubrication	Oil pressure, recovery cup
Degraded environmental conditions	Cleaning, air renewal checks

The various solutions known to alleviate this seizure problem, depending on the possible causes, are as follows:

Table 10: Possible causes of seizure and solutions (74)

Possible causes	Possible solutions
Excessively moist granules	Optimising the drying process
Granule incorrectly lubricated	Change lubricant
Granule too coarse	Reduce the size of the aggregate by adding fines
Excessively abrasive granules	Checking the condition of dies and punches Polishing tips Surface coating solutions for punches and dies
Defects in matrices	Check condition Polishing dies Examine other materials or surface coating solutions for dies
High compression force	Reducing force

2.2.5- Bonding

A recent study by Chattoraj S et al, highlighted the different techniques for solving the problem of sticking, which are internal and external lubrication.

Internal lubrication in tablet manufacture is deficient, adversely affecting final product properties such as mechanical strength and dissolution times. These adverse effects are related to the mechanism, quantity and incorporation of the lubricant, exemplified by MgSt. However, problems arise with under-lubrication, compromising lubricating properties and causing compression difficulties. Over-lubrication improves the lubricating properties but affects the quality of the final product. Finding the optimum balance of quantity, intensity and mixing time remains a challenge, making internal lubrication complex. External lubrication is emerging as an alternative, aiming to deliver the necessary quantity only at the interface between the particles and the tool walls, reducing friction without compromising internal cohesion.

Promising results then led to the development of several external lubrication systems, now offered by various companies, such as the PKB-1, 2 and 3 systems from Fette. The principle behind all these systems remains the same, consisting of suspending a lubricating substance, usually MgSt powder, in compressed air, then continuously spraying this substance onto the tool surfaces via a dedicated nozzle. The advantages of external lubrication are many, including reducing sticking during compression, improving the mechanical strength of the compacts and shortening their dissolution and disintegration times. However, despite these advantages, external lubrication has its drawbacks, such as high cost, complexity of implementation, regulatory requirements and a lack of in-depth scientific data. The performance of external lubrication in terms of ejection force reduction is also criticised by some, and the lack of in-depth studies on this technique is an obstacle to its development. Despite these challenges, external lubrication remains an interesting prospect for improving compression processes in the manufacture of pharmaceutical tablets.

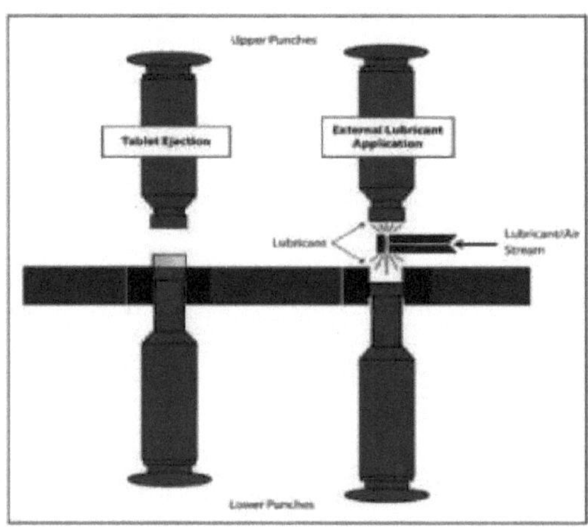

Figure 71: Diagram of an external lubrication system (135)

More specifically, for the different sticking variables mentioned above, a recent study proved that Sticking is a multifactorial phenomenon, originating from APIs, as well as formulation parameters involving active ingredients and excipients, and consequently, possible solutions are of diverse origins in the absence of a radical solution (120).

Table 11: Possible causes of sticking and solutions (74)

Possible causes	Possible solutions
Excessively moist granules	Optimising the drying process
Granule incorrectly lubricated	Change lubricant
Excess binder	Reduce the amount of binder Use another binder with a viscosity less
Hygroscopic material	Check the formula Check manufacturing and storage conditions

	Add an absorbent agent
Excessive concavity of the fists	Checking fist design
Low compression force	Increase compression pressure
	Reduce machine speed

With regard to picking, results from the literature have shown that by modifying the cutting angles in the raised letters and numbers on the compression tools, and by optimising the formulation process variables, a robust and reproducible region of the process could be identified to produce tablets of acceptable quality while avoiding increasing concentrations of magnesium stearate in the formulation (136).

Table 12: Possible causes of picking and solutions (74)

Possible causes	**Possible solutions**
Excessively moist granules	Optimising the drying process
Granule incorrectly lubricated	Change lubricant
Low melting point of raw materials	Using raw materials that raise the melting point
	Use lubricants with a high melting point
High proportion of binder or excessively viscous binder	Check the formula
	Controlling manufacturing and storage conditions
	Add an absorbent
Pellet too hot for compression	Cooling the pellets and the compression machine
Defects in the head of the fistons	Check condition
	Fist polishing
	Surface coating solutions for fistons
Poor condition of the engraving on the knuckles	Avoid engravings or make them as large as possible
Low compression force	Increase compression force

2.3- Deployment of a new control strategy

Pharmaceutical compression is the manufacturing stage most subject to IPC, so some checks are carried out at the beginning and end of the batch, others after each change of team, but also during manufacture with a high frequency that differs from one industry to another (usually every 15 to 30 minutes). These checks generally concern the measurement of thickness, average mass and hardness.

In order to increase yield, reduce labour costs and enable the operator to focus more on the appearance of the tablets produced, in other words, an operator could control two tablet presses as mentioned above, while reducing the number of tablets destroyed during the various tests to improve yield, reducing the frequency of these tests seems to be a possible solution.

One study (137) has shown that the state or frequency of control during compression is independent of product quality, the general definition of control state in ICH Q10 is understood to have the practical implication that when a process is in a state of control, past results are predictive of future results, and that these results will fall within a well-defined statistical distribution, often but not necessarily normally distributed. Although processes in a state of control often produce a high percentage of products within specified limits, this is not always the case, as the state of control is independent of product quality assurance. In other words, a process in a state of control will always produce a product that falls within a well-defined statistical distribution, although the tails of this distribution may eventually fall outside acceptable quality limits, at the expense of the quality assurance of the product.

he probability of a process reaching the specified limits is conveniently described by the process capability index (Cpk). In general, scientists often look for a Cpk > 1.33, which predicts a defect rate of less than 64 ppm due to the variability of common causes. Continuous processes are generally data rich and, as a result, care should be taken to avoid over-interpretation of individual data points, as values above specified batch average limits are likely to be observed even for processes capable under a controlled state, This is the case with the hardness test, since the aim is not to obtain a target value but rather an interval, and the distribution of the points is not homogeneous, adding to this the various regulation procedures specific to tablet presses, which make it possible to detect any tablets produced outside the required specifications and to avoid any possible deviation (77).

What is a robust process?

The aim of a capability study is to check whether a process is capable of generating performance in line with the expected quality. In the context of a capability study for a given process, the tolerance interval is compared with the dispersion, i.e. the agreement between the required performance and that actually obtained.

The tolerance interval is defined as the distance between the upper and lower tolerances. If the values obtained from the samples exceed these tolerances, the samples are considered to be non-compliant. This theoretical range, within which the parameter must evolve, is generally determined by the development department during the galenical development and feasibility study phases. By way of example, the tolerance range corresponds to the standards specified in the Marketing Authorisation Application (MAA).

The dispersion of the process is determined by calculating the standard deviation of the parameter under study. Ideally, the distribution of this parameter follows a Gaussian distribution centred on the mean value, and the standard deviation is correctly controlled. The dispersion at 'six standard deviations' (60) encompasses the interval containing 99.73% of the values of the parameter under study. In other words, the probability of finding a value between plus or minus three standard deviations is 0.9973, or 99.73% (138).

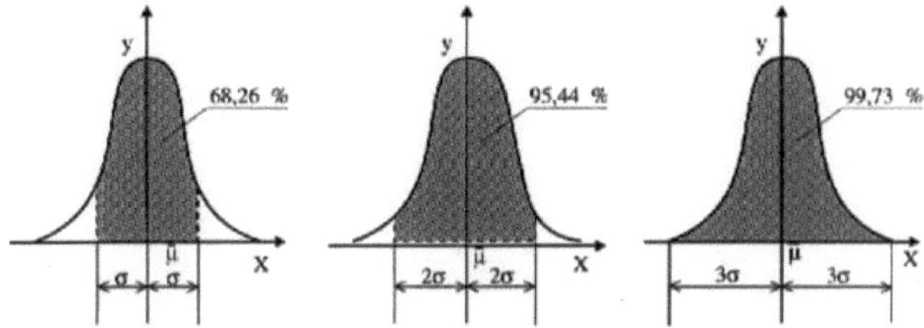

Figure 72: Dispersion at six standard deviations (139)

As the dispersion of the parameter is reduced, the standard deviation is reduced proportionally, which means that the risk of exceeding tolerances is reduced. In other words, a reduction in standard deviation is synonymous with production conformity.

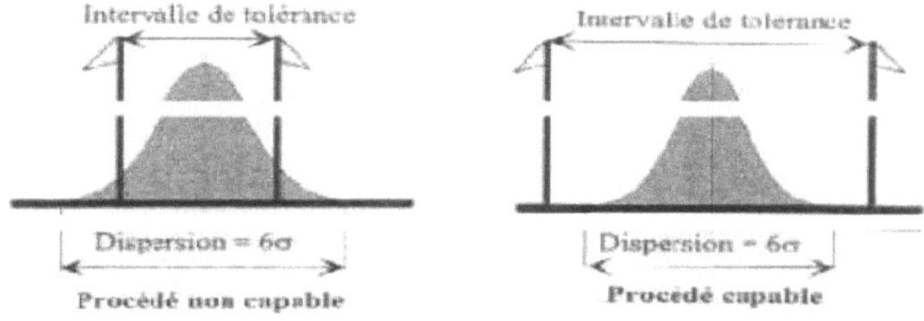

Figure 73: Capability of two processes with regard to the tolerance interval and dispersion (139)

The graphical representation highlights the distinction between a non-capable and a capable process:
•	In the first case, the process has a dispersion that exceeds the tolerances, resulting in a certain percentage of non-compliant production.
•	On the other hand, the second process is characterised by a dispersion that remains within the tolerance range, thus ensuring complete conformity of the production.
Based on the tolerance interval and dispersion, two types of capability are studied:
•	Potential" capability
•	Real" capability

- Potential capacity :

95

The potential capability (Cp) compares the tolerance interval (IT) of the specifications with the dispersion of the process. The formula for calculating this capability is as follows (140):

$$Cp = \frac{Intervalle\ de\ tolérance}{Dispersion} = \frac{IT}{6\sigma}$$

The interpretation of the capability studies is summarised in the table below:

Table 13: Interpretation of different capability values (139)

IT	Cp<0.67	0.67<Cp< 1.00	1.00<Cp<1.33	1.33< Cp<1.67	1.67< Cp< 2.00	Cp>2.00
6a	Very bad	Wrong	Very average	Average	Good	Tres good

A process is considered suitable or "capable" when its dispersion remains below 75% of the tolerance interval, which is reflected by a Cp index greater than 1.33.

- Real capability:

The aim of actual capability is to assess how closely the process is aligned with the expected target value. Calculating potential capability is not sufficient to characterise the performance of a process. The study of potential capability does not reflect the central tendency of the process, as two processes with identical dispersion may occupy different positions within the tolerance interval (141).

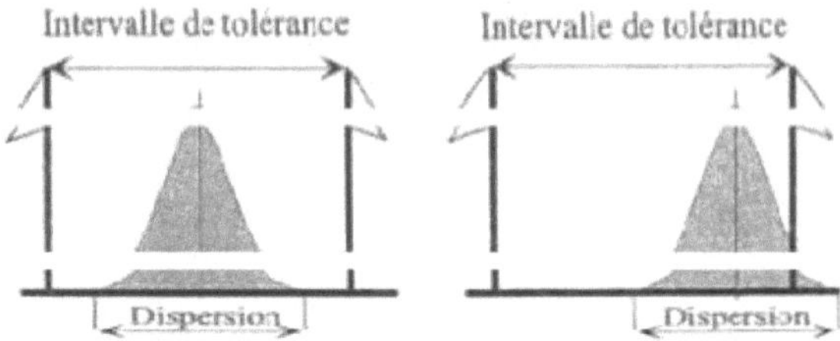

Figure 74: Capability of two processes in relation to their centring (139)

The first process is centred, while the second is decentred, yet their potential capacities are comparable due to their identical dispersions. In these two situations, the risk of producing results outside the norm, i.e. outside the tolerance limits, is different. This is why it is essential to introduce another indicator, the real capacity, rated Cpk, which takes into account the centring of the process.

$$Cpk = \frac{Distance\ (moyenne-limite\ la\ plus\ proche)}{\frac{1}{2}\ de\ la\ Dispersion}$$

C k = *Distance (mean - nearest limit') - of the Dispersion*

When the Cp and Cpk indicators are identical, the process is perfectly centred on the target value (141).

As a result, a risk analysis could be carried out to determine whether this theory could be applied to tablet presses, thereby reducing the number of IPCs during compression and optimising production by reducing the number of tablets destroyed without affecting the final quality of the tablet. A similar approach was carried out on distribution and packaging lines (142) using the FMECA approach and showed that it was possible to check at a lower frequency without risk of impacting the quality of the blisters produced. This approach could be applied to a compression line using the same approach in different pharmaceutical industries.

3- Artificial intelligence and pharmaceutical production

3.1- Optimising a process with AI

The transition to digital production offers the potential for significant improvements in productivity and the robustness of processes and equipment, in addition to activity forecasting and planning. It is based on the integration of sensors and connected objects that collect data in real time from operations in progress and previous batches. This data is then centralised in dedicated systems for real-time collection and analysis. This approach enables in-depth analysis, realistic forecasts and more effective process control.

The rapid evolution of technological tools is contributing to this transformation, with the emergence of ultra-fast processors, affordable and practical data storage solutions, and sophisticated analysis and control algorithms. These innovations provide organisations with a real-time view of their operations, giving them the flexibility to adapt to any potential drift in their processes (143).

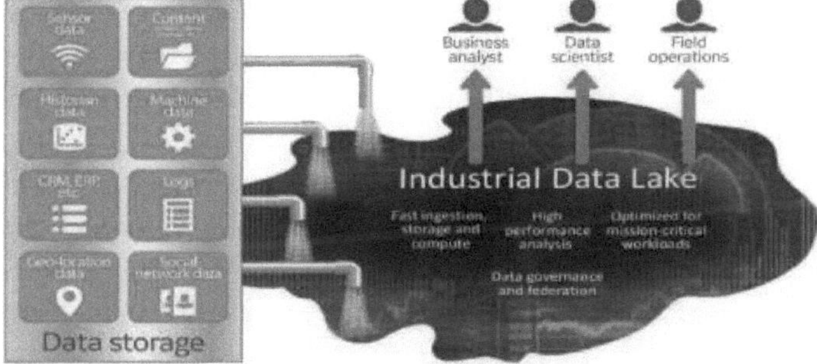

Figure 75: Diagram illustrating the Industrial Data Lake concept (143)

The data will come from a multitude of sources, such as sensors, historical data, information from machines, software packages, and so on. This data will be brought together in an 'industrial data lake', requiring significant storage, analysis and calculation capacity. Various types of information can be extracted from this data lake, particularly for managers, who will be able to monitor production rates, identify bottlenecks and track downtime, among other things.

One example of such a solution is Cytiva Digital's Predix platform (144). This platform continuously collects information using sensors, stores it in the cloud and then analyses it to provide a control and process improvement platform for drug manufacturers. The aim is to significantly reduce stocks and maintenance costs, relieve computer systems of ancillary tasks and concentrate on core activities, while complying with legislation on data storage. Reckitt Benckiser and Lek Pharmaceuticals have already adopted this solution to monitor and optimise their processes.

Artificial intelligence (AI) will also enable the rigorous automation of certain repetitive production tasks, guaranteeing continuous quality by limiting the biases associated with human intervention. It will direct the human workforce towards more complex activities with higher added value (145).

If we envisage almost total automation of production, a machine will be able to analyse a digital purchase order, plan production, order the necessary materials, monitor and manage manufacture, packaging, storage and finally dispatch of the product to the customer. The benefits of this approach are manifold: more efficient use of materials and raw materials, faster and more efficient production, and constant compliance with critical quality attributes, which must lie within a range of values to ensure the quality of the end product.

The detailed analysis of production stages, made possible by sensors, will make it possible to optimise various processes such as compression, granulation or chemical synthesis. This involves eliminating specific unnecessary operations or combining them using deep learning algorithms integrated into equipment capable of performing different tasks simultaneously (multi-tasking). In addition, analysis of the manufacturing attributes and product characteristics of each batch will enable selection of the manufacturing recipe offering the final dosage that best meets the specifications.

In conclusion, artificial intelligence (AI) offers a significant advance in optimising the many critical parameters of the compression process. By analysing data in real time and using complex algorithms, AI enables dynamic adaptation of compression, guaranteeing more accurate, efficient and compliant production. The integration of AI into pharmaceutical compression thus helps to increase tablet quality while optimising resources and enhancing the reliability of the process (146).

3.2- Real-time control of production parameters

The control of critical production parameters is closely linked to the optimisation of production processes, incorporating technologies such as the use of sensors to monitor variables in real time. This approach enables any deviation from the required specifications to be detected quickly, offering the opportunity to rectify the situation before thresholds are crossed at which the batch cannot be released.

Industries such as Novartis (147) have been experimenting with these technological advances on several sites, thereby enhancing the quality of pharmaceutical production. The monitoring of these parameters also extends to essential aspects such as water quality, which is widely used in production and equipment cleaning. The application of visual recognition technologies, such as SCADA (Supervisory Control And Data Acquisition) systems, enhances real-time predictive maintenance, minimising downtime through instant detection of faulty or worn parts, or one-off or recurring faults in manufactured products. Detection would be instantaneous, enabling reduced downtime and optimising yields in pharmaceutical production. This would result in a significant reduction in maintenance and production costs.

An analysis carried out by Siemens estimates that it can reduce downtime by up to 30% by digitising production lines (148).

3.3- Risk management

Risk management is an essential step within quality management systems, aimed at ensuring patient safety. ICH Q9 (149), on risk management, incorporates various phases in this process, including identification, analysis, evaluation, control (by acceptance or reduction of the risk) and finally periodic re-evaluation of these risks.

Risk identification is based on extensive databases created and maintained from process parameters, machine configurations and historical data on previous situations. An AI tool for integrated risk management can thus draw up a complete map of the risks specific to the company, analyse them and suggest corrective and preventive measures to avoid them. Thanks to AI, decision trees specific to each risk situation are drawn up, recommending the solution offering the highest probability of achieving a 'zero' risk level, presented in the form of dashboards. This model is regularly updated on the basis of current standards, internal procedures and other comprehensive and valid documents.

Risk analysis is frequently carried out manually, involving the management of a large volume of information. It can be difficult to establish links between situations that do not appear to be connected at first glance. Artificial intelligence eliminates this human bias, overcoming human limitations to better identify and anticipate risks. Risk analysis is often a time-consuming process, requiring the participation of a large number of people. Using AI software in this area helps to ensure regulatory compliance, save time, increase the robustness of processes and guarantee the quality of finished products (146).

4-Conclusion

In conclusion, current solutions to pharmaceutical compression problems have evolved considerably, incorporating innovative technologies to improve the efficiency, quality and cost-effectiveness of the process. Advances in compression equipment design, real-time quality control and the use of optimised formulations have helped to overcome some of the major challenges associated with pharmaceutical compression. Nevertheless, the lack of radical solutions to manufacturing problems remains a major handicap to manufacturers in coping with the losses they generate.

The outlook for the future is promising, with increasing emphasis on the integration of AI and advanced technologies such as these in pharmaceutical production. Advanced numerical simulation and full process automation thanks to AI pave the way for more efficient production and rapid adaptation to market changes.

General conclusion

Through this comprehensive manual, the careful identification of the critical parameters in the pharmaceutical compression process and the in-depth understanding of the interaction mechanisms with the tooling have not only shed light on the current challenges, but have also laid the foundations for a significant acceleration in the development of the process. By shedding light on these parameters, the research has provided invaluable keys to solving the problems encountered, while paving the way for strategic optimisation of various aspects of pharmaceutical compression.

The development of the compression process, as a crucial step in pharmaceutical production, will benefit tangibly from this in-depth understanding. The conclusions of this research are not only limited to the resolution of current problems, but also provide a solid basis for the continued improvement of the process. By adopting these discoveries, the pharmaceutical industry could envisage faster integration of new formulations, reducing the time needed to bring new products to market, but also speeding up the start-up of newly installed equipment.

In addition, solving current problems in pharmaceutical compression through a thorough understanding of the interactions with the tooling opens the door to further optimisation. This translates into improved yields, reduced raw material losses and better quality tablets. These improvements have direct implications for the profitability and competitiveness of pharmaceutical companies.

The way forward lies in the ongoing development of processes, products and equipment. Research has provided insights to guide these developments. The adoption of emerging technologies, such as the integration of artificial intelligence into process control, could play a key role in continuous optimisation. Similarly, the exploration of new materials for tooling could open up unprecedented avenues in terms of efficiency and durability.

By encouraging continuous development, this thesis proposes a roadmap for the pharmaceutical industry, calling for the implementation of agile research and development practices. By embracing a continuous improvement approach, companies can stay at the forefront of innovation, meet ever-changing regulatory requirements, and maintain a competitive position in the marketplace.

However, the lack of research into certain aspects of compression, and the failure to apply recent technologies such as artificial intelligence directly to the process, leaves a number of grey areas that should be clarified by encouraging scientific research in this area, but also by encouraging manufacturers to embrace change.

In conclusion, this book offers much more than simple problem solving, it offers a proactive and evolving vision for the future of pharmaceutical compression.

Resume

Title : Compression in the pharmaceutical industry: set-up parameters, interactions with tooling and process optimisation.

Author: Abdeldjalil Souheil MOUMENI.

Rapporteur: Prof. J.AKRIM

Key words: Pharmaceutical compression, tablets, punches, dies, rotary presses.

General introduction: This manual focuses on pharmaceutical compression, aiming to synthesise recent research in order to optimise industrial processes, particularly when integrating new equipment. It seeks to solve current challenges and improve the efficiency of tablet production by taking account of technological advances.

Chapter 1: The first chapter provides a comprehensive overview of pharmaceutical compression, covering topics ranging from basic definitions to the steps involved in the compression process. It explores compressibility criteria, the cohesive mechanisms of compression and the different types of deformation possible. Highlighting specific cases such as direct compression, the chapter also emphasises the importance of quality control in ensuring the conformance of compresses.

Chapter 2: Chapter Two looks in detail at the equipment and techniques employed in pharmaceutical compression, with particular emphasis on reciprocating and rotary machines. It assesses the advantages and disadvantages of each type of machine, as well as the principles of primary and secondary control. In addition, it examines tooling and accessories such as metal detectors and dust collectors, highlighting the importance of equipment qualification in ensuring the correct operation and quality of tablets.

Chapter 3: The third chapter focuses on the fundamental parameters of the pharmaceutical compression process, highlighting the concept of QBD and analysing the formulation, technological and operating parameters in detail. It covers the characterisation of raw materials, the influence of excipients, and the importance of the shape and integrity of the tooling, as well as the determination of operating parameters. The maintenance and customisation aspects of the equipment are also highlighted to ensure tablet quality.

Chapter 4: The final chapter explores interactions with tooling and pharmaceutical compression defects, proposing solutions and strategies to improve tablet press performance. It also examines the role of artificial intelligence in optimising pharmaceutical processes, highlighting its impact on production quality and efficiency.

Overall conclusion: This handbook on pharmaceutical compression examines the key parameters, catalysing industrial advancement. It offers resolutions and improvement tactics for companies, while emphasising the need for continued research and adoption of new technologies to maintain competitiveness.

Summary

Title : Pharmaceutical Compression: Development Parameters, Tooling Interactions, and Process Optimization.

Author : Abdeldjalil Souheil MOUMENI

Supervisor : Prof. J.AKRIM

Keywords : Pharmaceutical compression, tablets, punches, dies, rotary presses.

General Introduction : This book focuses on pharmaceutical compression, aiming to synthesize recent research to optimize industrial processes, particularly during the integration of new equipment. It seeks to address current challenges and enhance tablet production efficiency while considering technological advancements.

Chapter 1: The first chapter provides a comprehensive overview of pharmaceutical compression, covering topics ranging from basic definitions to the stages of the compression process. It explores compressibility criteria, tablet cohesion mechanisms, and various types of possible deformations. By highlighting specific cases such as direct compression, the chapter also emphasizes the importance of quality controls to ensure tablet compliance.

Chapter 2 : The second chapter delves into the equipment and techniques used in pharmaceutical compression, focusing on alternative and rotary machines. It evaluates the advantages and disadvantages of each machine type, as well as primary and secondary regulation principles. Additionally, it examines tooling elements and accessories such as metal detectors and dust collectors, underscoring the importance of equipment qualification to ensure proper functioning and tablet quality.

Chapter 3 : The third chapter concentrates on the fundamental parameters of the pharmaceutical compression process, highlighting the Quality by Design (QBD) concept and analyzing formulation, technological, and operational parameters in detail. It addresses raw material characterization, the influence of excipients, and the importance of tooling shape and integrity, as well as the determination of operational parameters. Maintenance and equipment customization aspects are also emphasized to ensure tablet quality.

Chapter 4 : The final chapter explores interactions with tooling and pharmaceutical compression defects, offering solutions and strategies to enhance tablet press performance. It also examines the role of artificial intelligence in optimizing pharmaceutical processes, underscoring its impact on production quality and efficiency.

General Conclusion : This book on pharmaceutical compression scrutinizes key parameters, thereby catalyzing industrial advancement. It provides resolutions and improvement tactics for companies, while emphasizing the need to continue research and adopt new technologies to maintain competitiveness.

Bibliographic

1.   VIDAL [Internet]. [cÉlë 27 Jan 2024]. Les differentes formes de mëdicaments. Available from: https://www.vidal.fr/medicaments/utilisation/regles-bon-usage/formes-medicament.html

2.   Poirier JC, Halfmann T. Validation of a compression process. STP Pharma Prat Tech Regiementations. 7(5):356-9.

3.   G. Sheiber, Medicament: excellence industrielle et optimisation des couts, STP Pharma Pratiques, volume 15-n°6, page 439.

4.   Alain Le Hir, Jean-Claude Chaumeil, Denis Brossard. Abreges de pharmacie galenique.

5.   Dilip M. Parikh.Handbook of Pharmaceutical Granulation Technology.ISBN : 9780367334772.

6.   Sarkar S, Chaudhuri B. DEM modeling of high shear wet granulation of a simple system. Asian J Pharm Sci. May 2018;13(3):220-8.

7.   LAROUSSE. Larousse.fr: free online encyclopedia and dictionaries. In 2023.

8.   Busignies-Goddin V. Recherche de lois de mélange sur des propriétés mecaniques.ISBN-13:978-613-1-50903-2.

9.   RIBET. 2003 Fonctionnalisation des excipients: application a la comprimabilite des celluloses et des saccharoses. These de Doctorat en Sciences Biologie Sante, Universite de Limoges, 263p.

10.   PSZCZOLINSKI.C. THE INFLUENCE OF THE NATURE OF THE BINDERS IN THE WET COMPRESSION PROCESS: CAS DU LACTOSE. UNIVERSITE DE LORRAINE; 2014.

11.   Chantraine F. Contribution a la solution des problemes poses par la présence de tensioactif au sein de compacts detergents. These de doctorat en Biologie Sciences Sante, Universite de Limoges, 214p.

12.   Moulay Saddik KADIRI. COMPRESSION DE POUDRES PHARMACEUTIQUES ET INTERACTION AVEC L'OUTILLAGE ANALYSE EXPERIMENTALE ET MODELISATION NUMERIQUE [These]. [L'INSTITUT NATIONAL POLYTECHNIQUE DE TOULOUSE];

13.   BOUVARD, D. Approches micromecaniques de la compression et du frittage des poudres Propos scientifiques, 2001 -I, n°26, 28-37.

14.   N'DRI-STEMPFER, B. Etude de 1 incidence des procëdës de granulation et de compression sur la couleur des compacts de poudres et de granums Thëse INPG & ENSMSE, Genie des procëdës, 2001.

15.   RENOUARD, M. De la particule au compact: vers une explication du phënomëne de clivage des comprimës de Paracëtamol.

16.   VAN DER VOORT MAARSCHALK, K. Stress relaxation of compacts produced from viscoelastic materials, Int. J. of Pharm. 1997, 151, 27-34.

17.   PORTAL, G. Analyse et optimisation du procëdë de compactage de poudres utilisëes dans les piles thermiques Thëse Universite Paul Sabatier de Toulouse, Sciences des matëriaux, 1999.

18.   LONG, W. M. Radial pressures in powder compaction Powder Metall, 1960, 6, 7386.

19.   LONG, W. M. Die design and related questions in powder compaction 2nd symposium of special ceramics, 1962, 327-340.

20.   MASTEAU, J.C. and THOMAS, G. Evolution and modelling of porosity and specific

surface area of pharmaceutical tablets during compaction,.

21.   TAKTAKJAMA, S. Contribution a l'etude du comportement en compression de poudres et de leurs melanges These de Lille 2, 1997.

22.   PONCHEL, G. La densification des poudres pharmaceutiques : fragmentation particulaire et compressibilite intrinseque These de doctorat, Univ. Paris-Sud, 1987.

23.   SCHMIDT, R. Comportement des materiaux dans les milieux biologiques Traite des materiaux 7, Presses Polytech. et Univ. Romandes, 1999.'.

24.   QELIK, M. Overview of compaction data analysis techniques Drug development and industrial pharmacy, 1992, 18 (6&7), 767-810.

25.   I. Saniocki, New Insights into Tablet Sticking: Characterization and Quantification of Sticking to Punch Surfaces during Tablet Manufacture by Direct Compaction, PhD Thesis, Hamburg University, 2014. https://ediss.sub.uni-hamburg.de/handle/ediss/5620.

26.   A. Tita-Goldstein, Compression shaping of powders: influence of process and formulation for the control of use properties, PhD These, Universite de Lorraine, 2013.

27.   J. v. Thomas, Evaluation and study on the adhesion of powder onto punch faces during tablet compaction, MSc These, Drexel University, 2015.

28.   Picart L. Resistance mecanique des comprimes pharmaceutiques tab-in-tab : caracterisation et lien avec les parametres materiaux et procedes [Internet] [phdthesis]. Universite de Bordeaux; 2022 [cite 7 dĕc 2023]. Available at: https://theses.hal.science/tel-03960044

29.   Florence E. Elasticite, course notes. [Internet]. [cite 10 fevr 2024]. Available from: https://fluides-complexes.fr/wp-content/uploads/2017/03/Elasticite.pdf

30.   Thoorens G, Krier F, Leclercq B, Carlin B, Evrard B. Microcrystalline cellulose, a direct compression binder in a quality by design environment-A review. Int J Pharm. oct 2014;473(1-2):64-72.

31.   de Craen AJ, Roos PJ, Leonard de Vries A, Kleijnen J. Effect of colour of drugs: systematic review of perceived effect of drugs and of their effectiveness. BMJ. 21 Dec 1996;313(7072):1624-6.

32.   BOUCHET-MATHIOU A. LA DEBLISTERISATION EN INDUSTRIE PHARMACEUTIQUE. UNIVERSITE CLERMONT AUVERGNE UFR DE PHARMACIE; 2022.

33.   Blicharski T, Swiader K, Serefko A, Kulczycka-Mamona S, Kolodziejczyk M, Szopa A. Challenges in technology of bilayer and multi-layer tablets: a mini-review. Curr Issues Pharm Med Sci. 26 Dec 2019;32.

34.   Rowe JM, Nikfar F. Modeling approaches to multilayer tableting. In: Predictive Modeling of Pharmaceutical Unit Operations [Internet]. Elsevier; 2017 [cite 18 Jun 2023]. p. 229-51. Available from: https://linkinghub.elsevier.com/retrieve/pii/B9780081001547000090

35. Gonnet C. Les enjeux du renouvellement des equipements au sein d'une industrie pharmaceutique: l'exemple du changement d'un parc de presses a comprimes. Grenoble Alpes;

36.   European Pharmacopeia. 2.9.1. Disaggregation of tablets and capsules.

37.   Pharmacopeeeuropeenne   . 2.9.5. Mass uniformity of single-dose preparations.

38.   Pharmacopeeeuropeenne. 2.9.6. Uniformity of content of single-dose preparations.

39.   Pharmacopeeeuropeenne   . 2.9.7. Friability of uncoated tablets.

40.   Pharmacopeeeuropeenne   . 2.9.8. Resistance to tablet breakage.

41.   Academie Nationale de Pharmacie, 2017, Comprimeuse, [online]. Available from: https://dictionnaire.acadpharm.org/w/Comprimeuse. In.

42.   DEVAY, Attila. The Theory and Practice of Pharmaceutical Technology. Pecs: Pecs University of Pecs. Chap. 24, Tabletting, p. 389-426. 2013.

43.   ResearchGate [Internet]. [cited 6 august 2023]. Fig. 1.1 - Description of the different stages of a compression cycle... Available on: https://www.researchgate.net/figure/Description-des-differentes-etapes-dun-cycle-de-compression-a-froid-en-matrice_fig1_30517627

44.   FROGERAIS A. Un siecle de machines a fabriquer les comprimĕs.Fascicule N°2 Machines a comprimer alternative. 2016.

45.   M.E. AULTON and K. TAYLOR. Aulton's Pharmaceutics: The Design and Manufacture of Medicines. 2021. ISBN: 9780702081545.

46.   Fette Compacting [Internet]. 2021 [cite; 16 Jul 2023]. The i Series from Fette Compacting. Available from: https://www.fette-compacting.com/en/products-technologies/tablet-presses/i-series

47.   Korsch AG: X 3 [Internet]. [cite 16 Jul 2023]. Available from: https://www.korsch.com/fr/recherche-de-produits/detail-du-produit/pharma-nutraceuticals/x3

48. Hata CVX Triple Layer Tablet Press - Elizabeth - PDF Catalog | Technical Documentation | Brochure [Internet]. [cite 7 dec 2023]. Available from: https://pdf.medicalexpo.fr/pdf-en/elizabeth/hata-cvx-triple-layer-tablet-press/114048- 175437.html#open805766

49.   FETTE Compacting. Operating instruction,technical documentation, tablet press P 3030.

50.   Arnold T. Implementation of new compression points following problems with packaging thickness.

51.   What is a tablet press - Medical consultation - News - LeadTop Pharmaceutical Machinery China [Internet]. [cited 28 Jan 2024]. Available from: http://www.capsuletabletmachine.com/news/what-is-a-tablet-press-machine-42634591.html

52. Natoli D, Levin M, Tsygan L, Liu L. Chapter 32 - Development, Optimization, and Scale-up of Process Parameters: Tablet Compression. In: Qiu Y, Chen Y, Zhang GGZ, Liu L, Porter WR, eds. Developing Solid Oral Dosage Forms [Internet]. San Diego: Academic Press; 2009 [cite 18 Jan 2024]. p. 725-59. Available from: https://www.sciencedirect.com/science/article/pii/B9780444532428000321

53.   Levacher E. Bonnes pratiques d'utilisation des outillages de compression.ISBN-10, 2951253575.

54.   FARES G. APPROACH TO COMPRESSION OPTIMISATION IN THE PHARMACEUTICAL INDUSTRY.

55.   TRUSTAR Pharma Pack Equipment Co, Ltd [Internet]. [cited 16 Jul 2023]. Rotary tablet press: the ultimate guide - KNOWLEDGE. Available at: http://www.cofpack.com/info/rotary-tablet-press-the-ultimate-guide-38564507.html

56.   14:00-17:00. ISO. [cite 27 jan 2024]. ISO 18084:2011. Available from: https://www.iso.org/fr/standard/57880.html

57.   Punzones y matrices [Internet]. FarmaFix. [cite; 16 Jul 2023]. Available from: https://farmafix.com/listado-general/punzones-y-matrices/

58.   Types and classification of tablet press: Which tablet press should you buy? - KNOWLEDGE - TRUSTAR Pharma Pack Equipment Co, Ltd [Internet]. [cited 28 Jan 2024]. Available from: http://m.cofpack.com/info/types-classification- of-tablet-press-which-37146565.html

59.   Continuous manufacturing, new I series. [Internet]. [cited 28 Jan 2024]. Available from:

https://www.fette-compacting.com/fileadmin/user_upload/Downloads/WhatsNext_2022-1_EN.pdf

60.   Fist Matrix Segments - I Holland Ltd [Internet]. 2023 [cited 18 Jan 2024]. Available from: https://fr.tablettingscience.com/punches-dies-segments/

61.   Croquelois B. Behaviour at fracture of brittle heterogeneous materials: application to pharmaceutical tablets [These]. Universite de Bordeaux; 2020.

62.   Broschuere_STYL_one-Evo-ENG.pdf [Internet]. [cite 22 nov 2023]. Available from: https://www.solpharma.com/wp-content/uploads/2021/02/Broschuere_STYL_one-Evo-ENG.pdf

63.   Metal detector rejects metal impurities to maintain consistent pharmaceutical quality [Internet]. [cited 26 nov 2023]. Available from: https://www.techik.net/fr/news-detail-1048341

64.   Kramer KD601x compact dust collector and metal detector [Internet]. DARRON Pharma. [cited 29 Jan 2024]. Available from: https://www.darron.fr/kramer/depoussierage-de-comprimes/depoussiereur-comprimes/

65.   CKDE AVEK - Gravity metal detector by MDR d.o.o. | DirectIndustry [Internet]. [cited 26 nov 2023]. Available from: https://www.directindustry.fr/prod/mdr- doo/product-190340-1888632.html

66.   Kramer high-speed tablet dusters [Internet]. DARRON Pharma. [cited 28 Jan 2024]. Available from: https://www.darron.fr/kramer/depoussierage-de- tablets/dusters-for-tablets/

67.   Econo Flex - Dust collector for tablets by kg-pharma | MedicalExpo [Internet]. [cite 6 dec 2023]. Available from: https://www.medicalexpo.fr/prod/kg-pharma/product- 114057-1056023.html

68.   Tableting - Romaco [Internet]. [cite 30 dec 2023]. Available from: https://www.romaco.com/products/peripherals/tableting

69.   VEDRENNE V. Equipment qualification in a pharmaceutical production industry. UNIVERSITE CLAUDE BERNARD - LYON 1; 2019.

70.   Kechemir N. Validation d'un Procëdë de fabrication d'une forme sëche Lyrica® Gëlule,Master en Pharmacie Industrielle Option Production,Universite Aboubakr Belkai'd de Tlemcen [Internet]. Available from: http://dspace.univ-tlemcen.dz/bitstream/112/7030/1/Validation-dun-procede-defabrication-dune-forme-seche

71.   ANSM. Guide to Good Manufacturing Practices. ANSM, 2017.

72.   European Commission. EudraLex. Good Manufacturing Practice (GMP) guidelines. European Commission. (Volume 4).

73.   Global harmonisation and the ICH. Mëdicaments essentiels : Le point. n°30: 56. 2001.

74.   SALAZAR R. Apuntes sobre tecnolog^a farmacëutica: Problemas tecnologicos en la fabricacion de medicamentos. Barcelona: R. M. Macian. Chap. 3.4, Fallos debidos al formato (punzones y matrices), p. 124-129. 2015.

75.   Caire M. Application du " Quality by Design " dans un centre de dëveloppement industriel ,thèse de doctorat en pharmacie , Universite de limoges,. 2011.

76.   Clemence T. Validation des procédés de fabrication : nouvelles reglementations FDA-EMA et application industrielle de la vérification en continu des procedes. [S.l.]: [s.n.]; 2014. 1 vol (111 f.).

77.   Canada S. Guidance - Pharmaceutical Development ICH theme Q8(R2) [Internet]. 2016 [cited 10 feb 2024]. Available from: https://www.canada.ca/fr/sante- canada/services/drugs-health-products/drugs/applications-submissions/guidelines/international-conference-harmonisation/quality/pharmaceutical-development- theme.html

78.   Wehrle P. Pharmacie galenique : formulation et technologie pharmaceutique. ISBN: 978-2-224-03142-8.

79.   NETZSCH - Analyzing and Testing. Leading in Thermal Analysis, Rheology and Fire Testing [Internet]. [cite 10 fevr 2024]. Active Substance-Excipient Compatibility. Available at: https://analyzing-testing.netzsch.com/fr/training-know-how/glossaire/compatibilite-substance-active-excipient

80.   Merienne C. Mesure, caracterisation et prediction de la stabilite des medicaments.Sciences pharmaceutiques. University of Lyon, 2020.

81.   Yihong Qiu, Yisheng Chen, Geoff G.Z. Zhang,Developing Solid Oral Dosage Forms - 2nd Edition.ISBN: 9780128024478.

82.   Chimactiv - Ressources pëdagogiques numëriques interactives dans l'analyse chimique de milieux complexes [Internet]. [cË1ë 10 fëvr 2024]. Available from: https://chimactiv.agroparistech.fr/fr/bases/hplc/theorie-illustree/5

83.   Pharmaceutical Excipients [Internet]. [^Të 30 Jan 2024]. Available from: https://www.ingenieurs.com/documents/cours/excipients-pharmaceutiques-117.php

84.   Paul J Sheskey, Walter G Cook, Colin G Cable.Handbook Of Pharmaceutical Excipients. ISBN :9780857113757.

85.   Na A, Ga M. Quantitative assessment of factors contributing to mottling of colored tablets II: formulation variables. J Pharm Sci [Internet]. fëvr 1976 [ci!^ 21 nov 2023];65(2). Available from: https://pubmed.ncbi.nlm.nih.gov/1255449/

86.   Wl D, Wt G. Batch production of pharmaceutical granulations in a fluidized bed. I. Effects of process variables on physical properties of final granulation. J Pharm Sci [Internet]. dëc 1971 [cit^ 21 Nov 2023];60(12). Available from: https://pubmed.ncbi.nlm.nih.gov/5158010/

87.   T S, D J, A J. Effects of powder particle size and binder viscosity on intergranular and intragranular particle size heterogeneity during high shear granulation. Eur J Pharm Sci Off J Eur Fed Pharm Sci [Internet]. March 2004 [cite 21 nov 2023];21(4). Available at: https://pubmed.ncbi.nlm.nih.gov/14998584/

88.   Jn H, Mh R, V W. The mechanical properties of some binders used in tableting. J Pharm Pharmacol [Internet]. dëc 1974 [^11ë 21 Nov 2023];26 Suppl. Available from: https://pubmed.ncbi.nlm.nih.gov/4156733/

89.   Shangraw R, Demarest D. A SURVEY OF CURRENT INDUSTRIAL PRACTICES IN THE FORMULATION AND MANUFACTURE OF TABLETS AND CAPSULES. Pharm Technol [Internet]. 1993 [cit^ 21 Nov 2023]; Available from: https://www.semanticscholar.org/paper/A-SURVEY-OF-CURRENT-INDUSTRIAL-PRACTICES-IN-THE-AND-Shangraw-Demarest/1df3c52b874e156bcc2e998c4a43be19ef0b090e

90.   J H, A A, A L. Initial studies of water granulation of eight grades of hypromellose (HPMC). Int J Pharm [Internet]. 26 Apr 2006 [cit^ 21 Nov 2023];313(1 -2). Available from: https://pubmed.ncbi.nlm.nih.gov/16510256/

91.   Boniatti J, Pereira Cerqueira AL, de Souza AC, Drago Hoffmeister CR, da Costa MA, Prado LD, et al. Galenic approaches in troubleshooting of glibenclamide tablet adhesion in compression machine punches. Saudi Pharm J. 1 Nov 2014;22(5):445-53.

92.   Kirsch D. Fixing Tableting Problems. Pharm Technol [Internet]. 2 May 2015 [cite 16 July 2023];39(5). Available from: https://www.pharmtech.com/view/fixing-tableting-problems

93.   FRULEUX, R., 2018. Implementation of a training system in 1 pharmaceutical industry:

application to compression tutoring. These pour le diplome d'etat de docteur en pharmacie. Pharmaceutical sciences. Lille : Universite de Lille. 79p.

94. Kosindustry, 2016. Difference between Rotary Tablet Press and Single Punch Pill Press.

95. Techceuticals - Pharmaceutical Training & Troubleshooting [Internet]. [cite 19 jul 2023]. Techceuticals: Pharma Manufacturing Training and Equipment Experts. Available at: https://techceuticals.com/

96. FRULEUX R. Mise en place d'un systeme de formation dans l'industrie pharmaceutique : application au tutorat en compression. These for the state diploma of doctor of pharmacy. Pharmaceutical sciences. University of Lille;

97. Equipo Co, Ltd del paquete de TRUSTAR Pharma [Internet]. [cite 19 juill 2023]. China maquinaria de preparation farmaceutica, proveedores de maquinaria de embalaje farmaceutico, fabricantes, fabrica - TRUSTAR Pharma Pack Equipment Co, Ltd. Available on: http://www.trustarpack.com/

98. libro Dr.Salazar con registro UB-VF1 20-01-16.pdf [Internet]. [cite 20 Jul 2023]. Available from: https://diposit.ub.edu/dspace/bitstream/2445/68462/6/libro%20Dr.Salazar%20con%20registro%20UB-VF1%20%20%2020-01-16.pdf

99. Osamura T, Takeuchi Y, Onodera R, Kitamura M, Takahashi Y, Tahara K, et al. Prediction of effects of punch shapes on tableting failure by using a multi-functional singlepunch tablet press. Asian J Pharm Sci. 1 Sep 2017;12(5):412-7.

100. Picart L, Mazel V, Moulin A, Bourgeaux V, Tchoreloff P. Influence of the punch shape on the core and shell structure of press-coated tablets. Int J Pharm. 25 Jul 2022;623:121930.

101. Adamus S.A. [Internet]. [cited 25 Jul 2023]. Adamus - More than tooling. Available at: https://www.adamus.com.pl/en/

102. PharmaState, 2018. Pharma Industry Guidelines : Tooling for Tableting [online] [Internet]. [cited 3 Aug 2023]. Available from: http://ww25.pharmastate.blog/tooling-for-tableting/

103. Natoli, D. Scribd. [cite 6 aout 2023]. Article Tabletting Resolving Tablet DefectsTablet (Pharmacy) | Wear. Available on: https://www.scribd.com/document/352241815/Article-Tabletting-Resolving-Tablet-Defects

104. Equipo Co, Ltd del paquete de TRUSTAR Pharma [Internet]. [cited 6 august 2023]. Prensa rotatoria para tabletas: la grna definitiva - CONOCIMIENTOS - TRUSTAR Pharma Pack Equipment Co, Ltd. Available at: http://www.trustarpack.com/info/rotary-tablet- press-the-ultimate-guide-38411959.html

105. Natoli-Whitepaper_Understanding-Importance-Punch-Length-Cup-Depth.pdf [Internet]. [cited 6 august 2023]. Available from: https://dh4b13or2bqf5.cloudfront.net/uploads/2017/02/Natoli-Whitepaper_Understanding-Importance-Punch-Length-Cup-Depth.pdf

106. Michael, D. Tablet press operation sticking by Techceuticals - Issuu [Internet]. 2017 [cited 6 Aug 2023]. Available from: https://issuu.com/techceuticals/docs/tablet_press_operation_-_sticking.p

107. Anbalagan P, Heng PWS, Liew CV. Tablet compression tooling - Impact of punch face edge modification. Int J Pharm. May 2017;524(1 -2):373-81.

108. Anbalagan P, Sarkar S, Liew CV, Heng PWS. Influence of the Punch Head Design on the Physical Quality of Tablets Produced in a Rotary Press. J Pharm Sci. Jan 2017;106(1):356-65.

109.   Kowalski L. Study of the correlations between a compression simulator and an industrial compression press. This paper was submitted for the degree of Doctor of Pharmacy. Pharmaceutical sciences. Grenoble: Universite Grenoble Alpes. 95p. 2019;

110.   NATOLI D. Tooling for Pharmaceutical Processing. In: AUGSBURGER L.L., HOAG. S.W. Pharmaceutical dosage forms. Tablets. Volume 3: Manufacture and Process Control. 3rd ed. New York: Informa Healthcare, 2008, pp. 1-48. ISBN : 9781420063455.

111.   I Holland - Home - Comprims Science [Internet]. 2020 [cited 18 Jan 2024]. Available at: https://fr.tablettingscience.com/

112.   Kirsch Doug. Natoli Engineering, 2017. How does turret condition affect tablet production? Tablet & Capsules, Solid Dose Digest [Internet]. Available from: https://www.tabletscapsules.com

113.   Juan, A. Farmafix, Notas tecnicas. Cuando pulir las puntas de los punzones. Available at: https://farmafix.com

114.   C. Ouvrard, Optimisation des parametres de compression des procedes de fabrication du site Merck Sante de Semoy, dissertation, Faculte de pharmacie de Rouen, 2006.

115.   A. Perrin, La compression des poudres pharmaceutiques : etude des differents parametres de compression, thesis, Faculte de pharmacie de Lille, 2006.

116.   MORIN G. Manufacturing defects in tablets. PharmatermMD, Bulletin terminologique de l'industrie pharmaceutique, 2006, vol. 17, pp.1-6.

117.   ICH Q8 (R2) Pharmaceutical development - Scientific guideline | European Medicines Agency [Internet]. [cЛĕ 14 Jan 2024]. Available from: https://www.ema.europa.eu/en/ich-q8-r2-pharmaceutical-development-scientific-guideline

118.   CARDOT P. Spĕcificitĕs du marché pharmaceutique Japonais : exemple de 1 inspection automatique de comprimĕs.Thĕse pour obtenir le grade de DOCTEUR DE L'UNIVERSITE DE LIMOGES.

119.   VISUAL DEFECTS ON COMPROMISES: ZOOM ON THE CAUSES OF APPEARANCE [Internet]. Sensum - Computer Vision Systems. [cиĕ 21 Jan 2024]. Available from: https://www.sensum.eu/fr/posts/examen-des-motifs-dapparition-de-defauts- visuals-the-most-current-on-tablets/

120.   Chattoraj S, Daugherity P, McDermott T, Olsofsky A, Roth WJ, Tobyn M. Sticking and Picking in Pharmaceutical Tablet Compression: An IQ Consortium Review. J Pharm Sci. Sep 1, 2018;107(9):2267-82.

121.   Thomas JV. Evaluation and study on the adhesion of powder onto punch faces during tablet compaction [Internet] [Master of Science]. Drexel University; 2015 [cиĕ 13 Nov 2023]. Available from: https://ResearchDiscovery.drexel.edu/esploro/outputs/graduate/991014632836904721

122.   Li Z, Zhao L, Lin X, Shen L, Feng Y. Direct compaction: An update of materials, trouble-shooting, and application. Int J Pharm. 30 Aug 2017;529(1 -2):543-56.

123.   Costa NF, Paulo MG, Diogo HP, Pinto JF. Solving a sticking related tablet problem by multivariate statistics and computational tomographic analysis. Powder Technol. 1 May 2020;367:456-63.

124.   C. Al-Karawi. Multifactorial analyses of the sticking tendency of ibuprofen and ibuprofen sodium dihydrate tablet formulations, Thesis, Hamburg University, 2018.

125.   Tablet press operation sticking by Techceuticals - Issuu [Internet]. 2017 [cited 26 nov 2023]. Available from: https://issuu.com/techceuticals/docs/tablet_press_operation_-_sticking.p

126.   Manufacturing Chemist, 2017. "How to avoid sticking and picking" [Internet]. [cite 26 nov 2023]. Available from: https://www.manufacturingchemist.com/

127.   Kadiri MS. Compression of Pharmaceutical Powders Interaction with Tooling. ISBN-10: 6138410009.

128.   CLICOPHA [Internet]. [cite 30 dec 2023]. Available at: https://www.i2m.u-bordeaux.fr/Projets/Projets-ANR/CLICOPHA

129.   Lamination - acadpharm [Internet]. [cite; 4 fèvr 2024]. Available from: https://dictionnaire.acadpharm.org/w/index.php?title=Laminage&mobileaction=toggle_view_desktop

130.   Mazel V. Etude de la compression pharmaceutique a 1 aide d'une approche de mecanique des milieux continus [online]. Habilitation a diriger les recherches. Process engineering. University of Bordeaux. Chap. 3, 3 Application de la MEF pour la compréhension des phenomenes en cours de compression dans le cas des comprimes biconvexes, p. 50-65. Available at https://hal.archives-ouvertes.fr/tel-01963729/ [These]. 2018.

131.   Matt Bundenthal, May 2, 2017. "Optimizing Yields on Modern Tablet Presses," Pharmaceutical Technology-05-02-2017, Volume 41, Issue 5. Pages: 66-68, 71.

132.   Optimising the yield of a tablet press, Pharmtech, [Internet]. [cite 1 jan 2024]. Available from: https://www.pharmtech.com/view/optimizing-yields-modern- tablet-presses

133.   President FM. Pharma Manufacturing. 2021 [cite 1 jan 2024]. Optimising the efficiency of a tablet press, Pharma manufacturing. Available at: https://www.pharmamanufacturing.com/sector/small-molecule/article/11293042/back-to-basics-on-tablet-press-efficiency

134.   Basim P, Haware RV, Dave RH. Tablet capping predictions of model materials using multivariate approach. Int J Pharm. Oct 5, 2019;569:118548.

135.   Papp MK, Venkatesh G, Harmon T. Specialised techniques for developing odt dosage forms. ONdrugDelivery. 1 Jan 2010;8-10.

136.   Sabir A, Evans B, Jain S. Formulation and process optimization to eliminate picking from market image tablets. Int J Pharm. 14 March 2001;215(1):123-35.

137.   Almaya A, De Belder L, Meyer R, Nagapudi K, Lin HRH, Leavesley I, et al. Control Strategies for Drug Product Continuous Direct Compression-State of Control, Product Collection Strategies, and Startup/Shutdown Operations for the Production of Clinical Trial Materials and Commercial Products. J Pharm Sci. 1 Apr 2017;106(4):930-43.

138.   S99-223 GPF de Q* E medical devices and risk management - A standard X. Process validation: Cp,Cpk, standard deviation... statistical methods [Internet]. Qualitiso. 2019 [cited 4 fevr 2024]. Available from: https://www.qualitiso.com/cpk-capacite-fiabilite-process/

139.   Yekpe K. Linking material attributes and manufacturing process parameters to quality control testing, an application of the quality by design concept. 2014 [cite 19 dec 2023]; Available from: https://savoirs.usherbrooke.ca/handle/11143/5397

140.   Capability; potential (inside) for the function Normal capability analysis for several variables [Internet]. [cite 4 fevr 2024]. Available from: https://support.minitab.com/fr-fr/minitab/20/help-and-how-to/quality-and-process-improvement/capability-analysis/how-to/capability-analysis/normal-capability-analysis-for-multiple-variables/interpret-the-results/all-statistics-and-graphs/potential-within-capability/

141. Chap. 1 Capability of machines and processes. Available at: https://www.technologuepro.com/cours-

controle-quaite/chapitre-1-capabilite-machine-process.pdf

142.   Desirant J. Deploiement d'une nouvelle methodologie " In Process Control ' ' sur des lignes de repartition et conditionnement.

143.   Cytiva [Internet]. [cite 14 dec 2023]. Digital manufacturing of biologics. Available at: https://www.cytivalifesciences.com/en/us/solutions/bioprocessing/knowledge- center/digital-manufacturing-of-biologics

144.   New Predix Offering from GE Digital Brings Manufacturing Data to the Cloud | GE News [Internet]. [cite 14 dec 2023]. Available from: https://www.ge.com/news/press-releases/new-predix-offering-ge-digital-brings-manufacturing-data-cloud

145.   Harris Y. Improving workplace productivity with AI tools [Internet]. Powell Software. 2023 [cited 4 feb 2024]. Available from: https://powell-software.com/en/resources/blog/artificial-intelligence-productivity/

146.   HOERDT A. Artificial Intelligence and the Pharmaceutical Industry: New Challenges for New Innovations.

147.   GREF Bretagne [Internet]. 2023 [cite 15 dec 2023]. Pharmaceutical industry. Acceleration on big data and AI. Available at: https://www.gref-bretagne.com/resources/pharmaceutical-industry-acceleration-on-big-data-and-lia/

148.   Nouvelle L, Nouvelle L. L'Intelligence Artificielle : la solution a la productivite des entreprises pharmaceutiques - Augustin Marty. 10 dec 2018 [cite 15 dec 2023]; Available from: http://www.usinenouvelle.com/blogs/augustin-marty/l-intelligence-artificielle-la- solution-a-la-productivite-des-entreprises-pharmaceutiques.N780804

149.   ICH Q9 Quality risk management - Scientific guideline | European Medicines Agency [Internet]. [cite 15 dec 2023]. Available at: https://www.ema.europa.eu/en/ich-q9-quality- risk-management-scientific-guideline

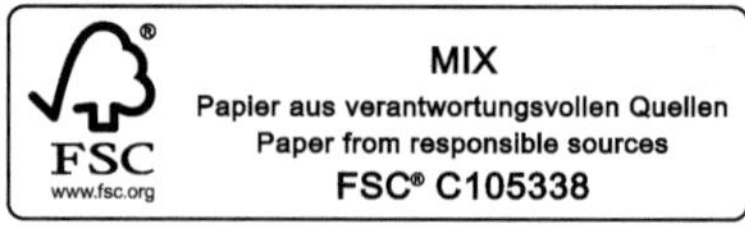

Printed by Books on Demand GmbH, Norderstedt / Germany